PAINLESS CHILDBIRTH

PAINLESS CHILDBIRTH
Psychoprophylactic Method

FERNAND LAMAZE

Translated by

L. R. CELESTIN
M.B., B.S., London
F.R.C.S., Edinburgh

HENRY REGNERY COMPANY · CHICAGO

First published in the English language in Great Britain in 1958.
Translated from *Qu'est-ce que l'accouchement sans douleur*?
Published in France.
© Editions La Farandole 1956.

Collaborators

René Angelergues
André Bourrel
Roger Hersilie
François Le Guay
Bernard Muldvorf
Pierre Vellay
Henri Vermorel

First published in the United States 1970 by Henry Regnery Company
114 West Illinois Street, Chicago, Illinois 60610
Manufactured in the United States of America
Library of Congress Catalog Card Number: 74-126152

TRANSLATOR'S PREFACE

MAN is the most versatile and least specialised of all the species in the animal kingdom. He has no special devices to swim, fly or run quickly. Yet he heads the primates.

The answer to this paradox is to be found in the opening lines of Pavlov's lectures on conditioned reflexes:* " The cerebral hemispheres stand out as the crowning achievement in the nervous development of the animal kingdom." It is the development of the brain that has given man the power of speech, and with it the ability to think, feel and act.

His bodily or endosomatic evolution may have stopped short of specialisation and robbed him of many physical attributes; but the appearance of his brain has given birth to a much more important form of evolution—that of the mechanical world within his reach, and sometimes called the exosomatic evolution. Here he has outstripped all the species of the animal kingdom and has achieved the highest speeds on land, sea or air.

If thought has offered him supremacy in the animal world it has also made him a prey to his own. His evolution towards a more comfortable civilisation has come to disturb his subconscious hold over himself and given the impression that he has lost his natural attributes. In fact, physically, man is now exactly what he was at the dawn of civilisation. But his emotions have changed; they have become complex and often made him suffer at the hands of his own species. No advancement in the exact sciences of physics, chemistry and (less so) of physiology, will afford any security against his emotions. Psychology and its sisters have still no great claim to exactness and do not often help him. Yet he would go a long way towards a world free from fear and apprehension if he knew more about himself.

* From a translation by G. V. Anrep.

5

Man's nagging enemy is the unknown. In the face of it the scientist is spurred to greater efforts; the curious are led to adventure, while the ignorant man (too often through no fault of his own) succumbs to his imagination.

Education is man's best friend in his struggle with the unknown, and it is my belief that an enlightened and prepared man is a better master of himself than one kept in the dark.

Sound and clear knowledge is less likely to create apprehension than mysteries and lack of information.

The patient is more intelligent than is normally realised, and will understand the nature of a disease or physiological process if properly explained. This was taught me dispassionately in the labour wards of my Alma Mater and I have had reason to believe it to be correct ever since. Furthermore, I feel that the patient should be offered, whenever possible, a generous explanation of the necessary treatment and care; it is, after all, a fair exchange for the trust placed in medical attendants; not to mention that health is a phenomenon of great social interest.

These are a few of the factors that have prompted me to undertake the translation of Dr. Lamaze's book, and it is my sincere hope that it will prove of some use in eradicating the worst example of the effect of the unknown, of perverted tradition, of misplaced morality and of ignorance in the mind of man—namely, that pain is a necessary accompaniment of childbirth.

L. R. C.

(Many footnotes and annotations have been included; they are mostly on technical terms that may not be known to some readers. Other notes are about men of science and topics which I feel may prove of some interest and create a pleasant digression. Additional diagrams have been inserted where it was felt they would make the text clearer.)

CONTENTS

FOREWORD

THIS book reflects the work carried out at the *Maternité du Métallurgiste* during some four years by a team under my direction.

Our never-ending anxiety has been to achieve an indissoluble unity by the constant sharing of our individual experiences and our views; in spite of this there has been no elimination of personality or any one point of view. We have approached the difficult problems that confronted us with the special knowledge acquired from our previous training and experience, and if we have always turned down narrow specialisation within the team, we each have, none the less, kept our own speciality.

It seemed to me essential that the concerns, ideas, and, to a certain extent, the style of each one of us should find their place in these pages. There follows, in consequence, some variety in the account; but I felt that this would not interfere with its well-founded unity.

Our work has diverse facets; it ranges from the practical tasks of organisation to those of providing educational classes for women, as well as the necessity for further theoretical studies of the still numerous problems remaining unsolved.

This diversity of character is frankly apparent in the book.

The first part is devoted to an account of the theoretical background that has made an effective fight against the pain of childbirth possible. This account may appear brain-racking to some; but we, too, have had to give much thought and reflection in our effort to assimilate Pavlov's theory. We felt that the omission of a true scientific account of the physiology of pain would not only create a serious gap capable of jeopardising the method we were propounding, but could have been taken as contempt for the reader on our part.

Let me ask those who may be put off by the specialised nature of the first chapters not to give up the book. They will, in the succeeding chapters, come across a style more familiar to them which will facilitate their going back to the previous chapters, if necessary.

The middle part of the book deals with the way future mothers are trained. There is nothing pompous about this training. It is simple and direct, and is more in the way of a chat than of a lecture. We have insisted on preserving its living nature, and this is why we have not hesitated to use the first person. We feel certain that the reader will find that this creates a better atmosphere for the exposition of the preparation for painless childbirth.

PREFACE

FOR millennia a curse has hung over mankind. Childbirth and pain appeared wedded for ever in close and mutually dependent bondage. No other fate seemed imaginable. So woman, fearful and resigned, passively consented to suffer the most exalting act in her life.

Everything has conspired towards this passiveness, this fear, this resignation. A fatalistic tradition handed on from generation to generation; ignorance of the most elementary physiological facts such as conception, pregnancy and childbirth (even sometimes fostered by forms of education); all these, aggravated by a false interpretation of the Bible, by stupid old wives' tales, by erroneous lectures, have engendered, out of nothing, the most favourable climate for the most alarming confusion. The resort to drugs of an analgesic, anaesthetic or amnesic nature to reduce or suppress pain in childbirth served only to strengthen in the minds of women the idea of this fatality of pain.

Symptoms were the sole concern; and doubtless with the most praiseworthy solicitude, medical treatments were multiplied, while women in labour were cared for in the same way as ill patients. What was really required was to go back to causes, to define the true and physiological nature of childbirth; and on that basis to work out the only suitable therapy.

This study of causes, their scientific determination and finally the redeeming solution, was the work of Bykov and his school, of Velvosky and of Nicolaiev, who started from the theory of the upper nervous activity elaborated by Ivan Pavlov during fifty years of experimental and clinical research.

The demonstration of the cortical nature of painful sensation and the mechanism of its transformation came from

11

the Pavlovian school. In 1912, as the result of researches done in Pavlov's laboratories, Mrs. N. Erofeeva had written a thesis demonstrating the conditioned character of painful sensation. She showed that pain is a cortical phenomenon, since the conditioned stimuli acted at cortical level and could be suppressed by the intervention of a new conditioning. Hers was a fundamental study and one can understand why it wrenched out of the English physiologist, Sherrington, the assenting exclamation: "Now I understand the psychology of martyrs!"

There is no need to say any more since the purpose of this book embodies a very full history of the psychoprophylactic method; but it is only fair to stress the role played by Velvosky in the application of Pavlov's theories to the psychoprophylaxis of pain in childbirth. It was as a neurologist at the clinics for railwaymen in Dniepropetrovsk that he started his first studies on this question as far back as 1920. It is fitting also to quote him when he states: " The teachings of Pavlov have strengthened the conviction that childbirth, in so far as it is a natural act, need not be accompanied by painful manifestations. We understood that pain in childbirth had not ' come to stay ', that it was by no means an attribute of the female sex and that it was not an unalterable and hereditary property. Hence the need not of trying to ' cure ' these pains or minimise them, but of explaining their causes, and from these to seek to *eradicate* them as acquired and generally accepted phenomena. We must conclude that parturition, which should be a natural and painless process, has become perverted. So we should try, not to cure the pain of childbirth by the use of drugs (since childbirth is not a disease), or inhibit it by means of hypnosis or suggestion, but to make every effort to destroy the concepts that breed this pain."

It was in the light of the experimental data of the materialistic physiology of Pavlov, that a precise, rational and safe method was elaborated. This method, applied without exception in all the lying-in establishments of Russia, made it possible for 86 to 92 per cent of Soviet women undergoing a normal labour to give birth without pain. The general application of the method was enforced by a decree from the Ministry of Health.

So, for the first time in world history, Soviet medicine set the improvement of conditions in childbirth as a national problem, as a problem of interest to the State.

Painless childbirth by the psychoprophylactic method is the result of the physical and psychological education of the pregnant woman during the last months of her gestation.

This physiological and experimental method aimed very definitely at abolishing the so-called unavoidable pain associated with uterine contraction during labour. It does not demand the use of drugs. There exists no contraindication of its use, and it carries with it no risk to mother or child.

This is, therefore, a well-defined entity, quite distinct from all the other methods advocated for painless childbirth. Its strength derives from its physiological bases. It has its measures of doctrine and technique, and these should be respected in order to ensure successful results.

It was in summer, 1951, that it was my privilege to witness, while on a medical visit to the Soviet Union, the application of the psychoprophylactic method. During tours that took me to Moscow, Georgia and Leningrad, I was able to investigate this new method on many occasions. I spoke to many obstetricians, I saw women during labour, and I questioned them after their delivery. Finally, in the unit of Professor A. Nicolaiev in Leningrad, I was present during a painless childbirth. Everywhere I witnessed the systematic application of the same method with results that were markedly consistent.

I had, at the time, thirty years of experience as an obstetrician. I had never been taught anything like this. I had

never seen it; nor had I ever thought it could be possible.
My emotional reaction was therefore all the stronger. I
made a clean sweep of all preconceived ideas and, now an
elderly schoolboy of sixty, I immediately decided to begin
studying this new science.

However tempting it was to reproduce such a method
and obtain such results, it seemed wise to me to take into
consideration the social conditions proper to each country.
In France, had the introduction of painless childbirth by
psychoprophylaxis been a faithful copy of the method
practised in the U.S.S.R., the results would have been un-
satisfactory. There were too many restrictive regulations
due to the different social climate and to financial difficulties. We had to work within the limits of reality, and it
must be admitted that our shortcomings were only too
obvious.

I decided, before anything else, to educate our women;
to inform them of the factual happening of painless childbirth in a great country. Then teach them, with the help of
unchallengeable proof, the correct, rational and unequi-
vocal character of that educational system that made it
possible for Soviet women to bring their children into the
world without this so-called " inevitable " pain. Finally,
by going into the how and why of things, to convince them
by using simple logic that French women too could enjoy
such good fortune.

Having instituted this favourable climate, I decided that
from the sixth month of pregnancy onwards (regardless of
the presentation of the child) all women under our care at
our Maternity Hospital would be prepared for painless
childbirth. Here I made a clean break with the practice in
the U.S.S.R., where the psychoprophylactic method was
offered solely to those with a normal presentation. This
was undoubtedly a great risk to take, but I felt that discrimination could lead women to entertain misgivings
about the method, and, for those who were not being pre-

pared, a still greater dread of childbirth. Furthermore, this gave us the advantage offered by mass discipline.

After a short clinical trial we decided to modify slightly the respiratory method adopted once the uterus went into labour. We have kept slow breathing during the first stage of labour, but taught rapid breathing during the second stage, and finally prescribed a panting type of breathing as the child's head presents itself at the vulvar orifice.

These were the basic foundations of the psychoprophylactic method for painless childbirth, as practised in France.

The only real difficulties we met all sprang from the financial problem with regard to accommodation, comfort and laboratories, as much as with the number and standard of the medical or nursing personnel. However relatively small our scheme, and modest our experience, we feel that it has, none the less, set an example.

My testing ground was the *Maternité du Métallurgiste* in Paris, which I had founded in 1947 under the patronage of my very great friend, Pierre Rougues. Then, with the help of a friendly team of doctors, midwives, physiotherapists and nurses, quickly raised to the pitch of my justified enthusiasm, and backed by the confident, firm and steady support of the *Union des Syndicats Métallurgistes de la Seine*, I was able to introduce in France the psychoprophylactic method of painless childbirth which I had witnessed in the Soviet Union.

With joy, but without surprise, I watched success crown our efforts. This will always be the case each time an enthusiastic team of doctors and midwives—whatever country they be in—undertakes to apply faithfully the Pavlovian principles of painless childbirth.

During a subsequent visit to the Soviet Union in February and March 1955, I was able to strengthen the knowledge I had received during my previous trip, and compare the results I had obtained during three and a half years with those being obtained in the U.S.S.R. at that time. I had the pleasure of seeing, and of hearing it said, that the method practised at the *Maternité du Métallurgiste* agreed basically with the Soviet method.

As Professor Malinovsky pointed out to me, it was not a question of contributing to obstetrical analgesia, but of introducing a method which is and which must remain the very basis of obstetrics.

It is of universal value. There is no question of difference between races. A woman is a woman regardless of her nationality or colour. In 1953, while on a visit to China, where the method of painless childbirth was being nationally instituted, my friend Doctor Vellay saw (in maternity hospitals in Shanghai appropriately equipped for the method) Chinese women give birth without pain; in maternity hospitals not yet so equipped women of the very same China suffered the pangs of childbirth in pain.

So it is not a question of a miracle, nor of illusion or subterfuge. A woman learns how to give birth, in the same way that she learns how to swim, or write or read; and she does so without pain.

In this essential education there is every reason to stress the determining part played by language and by speech as a physiological and therapeutic factor. Pavlov termed speech the second system of signalisation. Speech is the best means we have to prepare a woman for childbirth. By using words as the strongest stimuli at his disposal, the obstetrician fashions in the pregnant woman new conditioned reflexes with a view to suppressing painful reactions (Platonov, Chichkova).

This stresses the need to educate the pregnant woman and improve her knowledge; but more than that the teacher should constantly seek to improve his own knowledge. For this reason, medical men and midwives concerned with the realisation of painless childbirth have the imperative and vital task of unrelentingly improving their minds at the same time as making it their duty to act as dispassionate critics of each other.

In the same way, one cannot say too often to women that painless childbirth by psychoprophylaxis is not synonymous with laziness. André Bourrel in his lectures rightly keeps on repeating that " childbirth without pain is not childbirth without effort ".

This is a fundamental fact, and a woman must be imbued with the thought that she is essentially responsible for the success or failure of her own childbirth. No doubt, when the time comes, she will have at her side the watchful care she has been promised and to which she is entitled; but she must not cease to be the force which directs, controls and regulates her labour. Her mind, carefully educated, steadfast and alert, will know how to abolish pain. In the same way, it can magnify pain if misfortune or negligence decrees that she should fail in her task. Besides, the woman will be amply rewarded for her efforts by the inexpressible joy of having contributed enormously to the birth of her child, of being the first to cast eyes on its puckered features and to hear its first cry.

A woman who gave birth without pain has been able to describe perfectly what she felt. She writes: " I gave birth to Thomas by the psychoprophylactic method called childbirth without pain. When friends say to me, ' Well, did you feel nothing? ' I reply, ' Quite the opposite, I felt everything, and that is the wonderful part of it . . . the amazing experience in which each second has remained imprinted on my memory and in which pain has simply found no place.' "

The purpose of this book is to bring to the notice of the public a method of childbirth that has stood the test of time. Critics of the method cannot refute the manifest truth of the three following observations: first, that painless childbirth exists; secondly, that it springs from Pavlovian concepts; thirdly, that its general application has no limits. The seven hundred thousand painless deliveries of which the Chinese can boast have the value of undeniable proof.

It follows that if honest criticisms exist they will be proved invalid. One may ignore painless childbirth, but one cannot deny its existence. The interest it has aroused in the whole world is cogent. The moving enrolment of women and the ever-increasing interest of public authorities in France will help, no doubt, the extension, on a rational scale, of a method which will radically alter the fate of women throughout the world.

Dr. Fernand Lamaze

PART I

THE HISTORICAL BACKGROUND OF CHILDBIRTH WITHOUT PAIN

CHAPTER I

HYPNOSIS AND VERBAL SUGGESTION

PAINLESSNESS in childbirth resulted from the work of
Velvosky, Platonov, Ploticher and Changom seeking, for
many years, to solve the problem of eliminating suffering
during labour by applying the physiological concepts of
Pavlov.* The final understanding of psychoprophylaxis is
the result of lengthy research which covers two distinct
periods: (*a*) the use of hypnosis and verbal suggestion;
(*b*) the evolution of the psychoprophylactic method proper.

*The practice of hypnosis differs markedly from that of
psychoprophylaxis.* Painless childbirth had been achieved
by hypnotic methods as far back as the nineteenth century,
and such methods must be recorded as the first step in the
fight against the pain associated with childbirth. But to
understand the development of this totally new method of
psychoprophylaxis in bringing about a delivery free from
unnecessary pain one must first appreciate the shortcomings of hypnosis and the pioneer work of the Pavlovian
school on the nature and origin of pain—as well as the part
played by the spoken word as a physiological and therapeutic agent.

When hypnosis was still cloaked in its magic garb, the
mesmerists of old, through relying on the properties of
their so-called " medium ", had nevertheless noticed that
they could numb the senses of women in labour by inducing them into a hypnotic trance. Gerlin in Berlin, and
Lafontaine in Switzerland, had, as far back as 1840 and
1863 respectively, made it possible for childbirth to be
painless; but these were essentially selected chance cases.

About 1880 French physicians were using hypnosis as a

* Ivan Petrovich Pavlov: Russian physiologist of note, 1849–1936.

therapeutic agent. Charcot* had applied it at the Salpetrière Hospital in Paris; so had Bernheim in Nancy. They showed that there was nothing mysterious about hypnosis, and that one could give a rational explanation of it. Above all, they pointed out that it was possible to use it to induce a state of insensitivity that allowed operations to be performed, or labour to progress, without pain. Hypnosis had therefore graduated from its magical stage to its empirical one.

About the same time other French physicians practising hypnosis claimed similar successes; some quoted as many as ten cases in which complete insensitivity had been induced. Yet, in spite of these successes, hypnosis offered only a limited application and remained essentially empirical. No one could explain the mechanism whereby verbal suggestion influenced the hypnotised patient; nor were all cases successful. Another drawback was that the technical difficulties of its execution demanded not merely the skill of a qualified practitioner but, in fact, that of an expert.

All this does not rob such early practitioners of the glory of having been the first ones to attempt to render labour painless. On the contrary, they must be given their rightful rank as forebears in the evolution of the psychoprophylactic method.

Paul Joire of Lille, in 1899, went even further. From what must have been a limited experience, he ventured the following conclusions: " Pain is not an essential feature of delivery and serves no useful physiological function. . . . In fact it is not uncommon for contractions to start long before pain, and the first stage of labour is characterised by such painless contractions. This can be readily ascertained by laying a hand on the woman's abdomen;† as the uterus

---

* Jean Martin Charcot (1825–93): French neurologist known for his work on hypnotism and hysteria.

† Abdomen: that part of the body which lies between the chest and the groin.

contracts intermittently, its fundus* becomes firmer. In a similar way, by feeling the cervix† one notices that during a contraction the membranes become tenser and more obvious; yet it is only seconds later that the patient complains of pain—a further proof that pain and contraction are not related.

"Even when it has been demonstrated that pain and contraction are not related, some still argue that pain could play a useful part by stimulating new contractions, and so keep up (if not increase) the intensity of those already present. If this argument were correct, it would follow that by diminishing pain the contractions would decrease both in frequency and strength, and eventually the delivery would be slowed down. This does not stand examination. In the first instance, in a normal delivery without any external help, the most painful labours have not turned out to be the shortest; and conversely, those that have been slow have not been the least painful. In the second instance, in those deliveries made less painful by suggestion, and carefully and precisely observed, it has been our experience that, far from being slowed down, labour on the contrary has proceeded at a quicker pace in the majority of cases."

Joire was not unaware of the technical difficulties of hypnosis and therefore favoured the use of suggestion in the fully conscious patient. He would explain to her that she would feel contractions. These were the natural result of the useful efforts of the uterus as it was slowly expelling the child. They would cause her no trouble, nor would they be painful. He therefore further remarked: "Suggestion proved so effective that, as the head was being delivered, she mentioned calmly that she could feel the lips of the vagina being drawn apart, but that she felt no pain."

* Fundus: the rounded base of a hollow organ, remotest from its opening.
† Cervix: that part of the womb which encircles its opening.

Other countries followed suit. Kingsbury in England, Schrenk-Notzing in Germany and Pritzl in Austria advocated hypnosis. In Austria the practice of hypnosis led to a Congress on the subject at Innsbruck in 1922. By then hypnosis, which had originated in France, had been given up in that country. In Anglo-Saxon countries, however, it still found favour until quite recently amongst a few obstetricians applying it in an empirical fashion. In Russia it was used in 1880 by Dobrovolskaia, and at the Eighth Pirogov Congress of 1902, Matviev presented twenty-eight cases, in which twenty had responded successfully to the use of hypnosis. A further success was claimed by Niazemsky, and in spite of the efforts of Bechtchevev, who elucidated some of the aspects of hypnosis, the method progressed no further, remaining limited in its application and essentially empirical.

This stagnant attitude was suddenly galvanised into action by the changes brought about by the Soviet régime following 1917. New horizons were being opened to medicine in Russia; henceforth the prevailing system made it possible for a technique to be enforced on a large scale throughout the country. Pavlov received the full support of the State, and this enabled him to expand the field of his research and develop further his theory on the nervous activity of the higher centres of the brain.

By 1920 Pavlov had investigated the physiological background of hypnosis and had suggested a scientific explanation. He had exploded its hitherto mysterious nature and so made its elaboration and its application more possible. So, in 1923, one sees Platonov and Velvosky reporting to the Second Pan-Russian Congress of Psychiatrists and Neurologists on the use of hypno-suggestive analgesia in surgery, obstetrics, gynaecology and stomatology.* Platonov himself, in tackling the widespread application of hypnosis, sought the co-operation of obstetricians (Chesto-

---

* Stomatology: the study of diseases of the mouth.

phal, Syrkine, etc.) and before long the method found a place in the maternity centres of Kharkov. But it was left to Nicolaiev in 1927 to pioneer the application of hypnosis in obstetrics in the light of Pavlov's theories, and it was from that date that he and Platonov clearly demonstrated the importance of fighting fear in the parturient* by means of a psychotherapeutic approach. Several possibilities could be explored: one could either plunge the woman into a hypnotic sleep at the very moment of childbirth, or one could prepare her while under the influence of hypnosis, but allow her to come round for the birth—the hypnotist choosing whether to be present all the time or not. Yet another method was that of indirect suggestion; that is, an anaesthetic mask is used but no gas is made to flow through it. These various preparations of the future mother were carried out either individually or in groups.

Thanks to the improvements in techniques, and the rational manner in which they were applied, thanks to State help and to the propaganda carried out to bring these methods home to the public, it was possible to put into practice the concept of childbirth without pain in a great number of cases. In 1939, for example, Platonov, by applying various methods of suggestion, had a 65 per cent success rate in some 500 deliveries. Similar successes were claimed by Nicolaiev; while in Kiev, Syrkine taught 600 pregnant women this method with good results. The same picture was seen in Moscow, where Zoravomyslov used suggestion and published, in 1938, his results relating to 250 deliveries with no pain in 84 per cent of them. He used essentially a method of suggestion with the mother-to-be either hypnotised or fully awake. Subsequently he taught his method to some thousand women.

All in all, it is interesting to note that as far back as the 'thirties Soviet obstetricians, by applying Pavlov's principles (and through the nature of the prevailing régime)

* Parturient: an expectant woman at term (the time of delivery).

had managed to realise effectively, on a large scale, a method that abolished pain in childbirth.

Their experience had led them to conclude that such methods had no ill effects on mother or child, and that pain played no useful purpose whatsoever in childbirth.

From the practical standpoint their experience allowed them to be more precise about methods of collective preparation.

Nevertheless, hypnotic suggestion was not a reliable method for mass application. It failed to spread to the whole country. Its greatest pitfall lay in the fact that the subject played a passive role; though she yielded to various suggestions, it still happened that these suggestions remained coloured by the counter-effects of her past education, in which pain had always been associated with childbirth in some fatalistic manner for thousands of years. Hypnosis, therefore, was limited to the symptomatic treatment of pain in so far as it was held to be inevitable. It follows that more work had to be done along totally different lines to reach a complete solution of the problem of abolishing the belief that pain was a natural concomitant of childbirth.

CHAPTER II

RESEARCH ON ANTENATAL PREPARATION

MANY Soviet workers had stressed the importance of antenatal visits during which the future mothers would be made acquainted with the work going on in a maternity unit and the atmosphere that prevailed there. Furthermore, these women were given lectures on the various aspects of pregnancy and on the use of analgesia during delivery.

This concept of reducing or abolishing pain was already becoming an everyday topic of conversation amongst psychiatrists and obstetricians.

Skrobansky, in 1936, was of the opinion that it was important to impress on a woman the purpose of analgesia. He felt that a woman who had been made to understand the place of analgesia, and who felt confident, would benefit from whatever method was used; whereas a woman who was convinced that she would be in pain would feel pain regardless of the efficacy of the method used.

Malinovsky, on his side, was using various analgesic facilities extensively to fight the very idea of pain, while Nicolaiev in 1936 made the following statement: " Every obstetric hospital must popularise the use of analgesia in its maternity wards. Each woman who is ' booked ' in such a hospital must be told that other women in the same place are being delivered without suffering; she must get accustomed, from her very first visit, to the idea that delivery can be made painless; and when she is admitted it is not enough for her to know that painlessness is possible— she must actively see for herself. The obstetrician must induce in his patient a healthy frame of mind by remoulding her psyche already shaped by an education obsessed with the ancient belief that pain is inevitable." This remoulding

27

of the mind was insisted upon by Alexandrovsky and Iourievsky in 1939, in their attempt to obtain better analgesia.

In spite of all these individual efforts, the results fell short of what was expected. The methods used were not systematic, nor scientific enough. The psychoprophylactic approach will be proved to be something quite unrelated to hypnosis or to the above pattern of preparation.

CHAPTER III

THE WORK OF READ

ROUND about the same time, Grantly Dick-Read was studying in Birmingham the psychological factors responsible for the pain of childbirth, and was seeking to solve that problem.

His experience as an obstetrician had convinced him that the various analgesics so far used were inadequate, and he disputed the fact that they were without danger to mother or child. His opinion was that the emotional state of the patient could magnify enormously any pain which was present. He realised that there were unnecessary factors that could increase pain, and foremost amongst these were the lonely plight of the woman in labour, her ignorance of physiological processes, and the strangeness of the atmosphere of the maternity wards.

He also stressed the bad effects that resulted from fear born out of exaggerated old wives' tales, or those encountered in some books and newspapers—all making childbirth a bloodcurdling process.

In his book, *Natural Childbirth*, published in 1933, he advocates enlightening the patient so as to reduce or abolish fear, in addition to lectures on the various physical changes she is undergoing.

There is not the slightest doubt that Read's theories, at that time, marked an advance on the views then held on analgesia and constituted the initial effort towards a psychotherapeutic approach. Needless to say, his theories met with strong opposition both from the Britsh medical world and the Anglican Church and resulted in Read being shunned, if not abused.

His good work was unfortunately marred by a strong

empirical flavour and, in consequence, it failed to become accepted generally, and was for a long time practised by Read alone. As will be pointed out later, his theories lacked a sound physiological basis, and he was therefore at a loss to work out a coherent method that could be easily applied, or would sound convincing to most obstetricians.

Many years had to go by before childbirth without fear became common and effective practice in the hands of such eminent obstetricians as Professor Nixon in London, or Thoms and Goodrich in the U.S.A. The theories behind childbirth without fear have not progressed during the past twenty years and have hardly found a place in France, nor indeed have they undergone any improvement. It was not until the psychoprophylactic method was introduced that interest in it was stimulated. There is not a single publication in France, prior to 1951, which mentions the application of the theories of the Birmingham obstetrician. The way in which the public became infatuated with his doctrine stands in marked contrast to the lukewarm welcome Read had received in Paris only a few years previously.

Read's empirical work is of great interest, but it has undoubtedly been surpassed by the prospects of the psychoprophylactic approach.

CHAPTER IV

THE REALISATION OF THE
PSYCHOPROPHYLACTIC METHOD

THE second phase of the work of Platonov and Velvosky leads us to a new chapter in the history of obstetrical analgesia. Their observations on the shortcomings of hypnosis led them to the following conclusions:

(a) Pain had been found to serve no useful function and to be subject to the influence of the spoken word.

(b) Hypnotic methods had proved to be innocuous.

(c) Hypnosis could not be practised on a national scale; in fifteen years only eight thousand painless deliveries had been achieved; its application was essentially of an individual nature.

(d) Hypnosis required a well-trained staff and could not be made available to every practitioner or midwife.

(e) It was a therapeutic method that did no more than " treat " a pain looked upon as inevitable and essential.

(f) Finally, if straightforward suggestion could abolish pain, it was obvious that counter-suggestions emanating from the woman's environment and education could nullify the efforts of the obstetrician.

Platonov and Velvosky were led to hunt for the historical origin of the pain of childbirth and came to the conclusion that it had become a social phenomenon. Tradition, through the intermediary of speech so specific to the human race, had created and nurtured the fear of pain itself in the minds of women. The lack of knowledge of the future mother regarding the problems of childbirth turned her mind into a field fertile enough for the implantation of the exaggerated stories perpetuated by this tradition.

Platonov and Velvosky concluded that it was imperative to uproot the origin of this evil; that is to say, plan an education not only of the woman herself but of society as well, so that pain should be looked upon as unnecessary and useless, the aim of that education being to explode the dogma of inevitable pain, first in the mind of each expectant mother, and then on a scale involving the whole of society.

Instead of hypnosis and suggestion that concentrated on symptomatic treatment of the pain, Velvosky recommended a preventive training of the fully conscious woman by means of educational methods. *This approach appeals to the perceptive faculties of the woman, and makes her take an active part in her delivery, which remains under her control;* she develops by herself a fair number of contrivances that lead to the abolition of pain during labour. The ultimate aim of Platonov and Velvosky was, therefore, to refashion the attitude of women towards the pain of childbirth, to put an end to the fatalistic belief of pain as far as it is a social phenomenon, and to substantiate the opposite idea that pain is useless.

This is why this method of the prevention of pain through the use of words carries the name of psychoprophylaxis.

Platonov writes: " This question is settled once and for all by prophylactic transformation not only of the woman's attitude to pain, but of the attitude of society as a whole. It is achieved by education, not by treatment; by information and not by hypnosis or suggestion. It is the didactic method—the very soul of the psychoprophylactic approach —which will solve this problem. The pain of childbirth will disappear as a social evil, thanks not only to the efforts of medical men (of which we are but the vanguard) but more so by public influence and the efforts of educationalists and writers. The recasting of the mind is a very powerful instrument capable of altering unconditioned reactions, according to the law which states that ontogenesis* leads to phylogenesis."† However, it must be pointed out that these workers could not have brought forth such a new approach without the discoveries in physiology made by Pavlov. In fact to fight the presence of pain in childbirth, it was essential in the first instance to explain it scientifically, so that research had to be done to assess the following:

(a) *The part played by the cortex of the brain in the occurrence of pain.* Since 1912, Erofeeva had carried out a most important experiment, which became the starting point of childbirth without pain. She created a conditioned reflex by means of a painful stimulus and then converted it into a painless stimulus. She demonstrated that the cortex of the brain was able to repress real pain and, in no less a way, engender pain that has no actual distant starting point.

Bykov and his pupils Pchonick and Rogov studied thoroughly this question of painful conditioned reflex at a later date, and in 1949 Pchonick published an important document on this phenomenon.

(b) *The invalidity of the classical opinion that the uterus, like many other organs, has no communication with the central nervous system.* Without the presence of such communications between uterus and brain, it would be impossible to achieve a conscious control of delivery by the patient.

Pavlov had already shown that the brain could receive and analyse messages coming from viscera; and his pupil Bykov enlarged on this and published in 1947 in Moscow a book entitled *The Brain Cortex and Internal Organs.* This book did not fail to influence the work of Platonov and Velvosky, though, in fact, in 1930 and 1939 Kercheev had carried out important studies on the special problem of the relationship between the brain and the internal genital

---

* Ontogenesis: the evolution of the individual.
† Phylogenesis: the evolution of a race or group of people.

organs in animals as well as in women. Lotis in 1949 published, in an article on the same subject, the results of more precise experiments, and some of these will be referred to later. Airapetianz (1949) and Gambachidzé (1951) likewise devoted themselves to a study of genital interoception.

(*c*) Finally, one of the most delicate of all physiological problems was that of *the spoken word as a therapeutic factor*; in short, the physiological basis of psychotherapy. Here as well, the part played by the theories of Pavlov was of great importance.

As early as 1907 one of Pavlov's oldest pupils, Krasnogorsky, was investigating in his laboratory the peculiarities of the speech development of the child; his studies were to be followed by the publication of an important book in 1939.

Ivanov-Smolensky carried out, in both adult and child, many researches on the second system of recording reality—the use of speech. He had many followers amongst his pupils, and his work is one of the most important lines of development of Pavlovian physiology.

Platonov, too, made an original and fundamental contribution to the problem of the physiology of speech. Carrying on with the researches already mentioned, he published a series of works blazing the trail of a new formula which was eventually to culminate in the psychoprophylactic method. Thus, in 1933, he published *The Spoken Word as a Physiological and Therapeutic Agent*, and in 1936, at a conference on obstetrical analgesia at Stalino in the Dombass, he said: " Our ultimate end in the solution of obstetrical analgesia lies in the re-education and reshaping of a mental attitude in which for centuries a fatalistic belief in pain has found roots." In addition, in 1940, his work *The Problem of Psychotherapy in Obstetrics* was published in Moscow.

The very first physiological analysis of pain in childbirth was made by 1936 by Nicolaiev. It was subsequently elaborated by Velvosky and his collaborators.

Velvosky underlined the very important role played by the Pavlov Session of the Academy of Science of 1950 in the final adjustment of the psychoprophylactic method. The discussions at that Session established the value of materialistic ideas in biology and medicine and gave a new lease of life to the conclusions reached by Michurin and Pavlov in their research work. The name " psychoprophylaxis " was coined by Nicolaiev in 1949.

That same year Velvosky and his collaborators demonstrated their method and gave a preliminary communication on its efficiency during a meeting of obstetricians gathered at Kharkov.

In 1951 a conference on the use of analgesia in childbirth was held at Leningrad, under the auspices of the Academy of Medicine of the U.S.S.R. and of the Ministry of Public Health. Velvosky and Platonov, joined by Nicolaiev, explained the principles of the psychoprophylactic method and presented their results of its experimental application in Kharkov, Moscow and Leningrad. As all their results were very impressive, the Government of the Soviet Union decreed in July 1951 that the psychoprophylactic method should be applied in every maternity unit in the Union, from the biggest city to the most distant *kolkhoz* of Soviet Asia. So, for the first time in the history of medicine, an important discovery found widespread application in a vast territory only a few years after its elaboration.

In 1953, 300,000 deliveries were offered the benefit of this new method, with some 80 to 90 per cent success. The mass application of psychoprophylaxis has proved itself a workable proposition; and from the U.S.S.R. it has spread to surrounding countries. In China the method became common usage in many large cities as well as in the countryside after 1952, when several Chinese obstetricians paid a visit to the unit of Professor Nicolaiev in Leningrad. In 1955 the figure of 700,000 painless deliveries was given as the total so far reached.

Amongst other countries that adopted this method were the countries behind the Iron Curtain, France, other countries in Western Europe and North, South and Central America. In France it has been practised since 1952 in many towns, and some 10,000 painless deliveries have been recorded. Other Western European countries have taken it up and so have the Americans.

So the first stage has been reached in the dissemination of the psychoprophylactic method, which has proved not only of universal value but of such technical ease as to give equal success wherever applied.

Part II

WHAT IS CHILDBIRTH WITHOUT PAIN?

INTRODUCTION

In seeking to understand the significance of this historical background of the various methods of achieving obstetrical analgesia without drugs, one can demonstrate immediately how valuable and strongly scientific is the nature of the psychoprophylactic method of childbirth without pain; in a similar manner one can draw attention to its originality.

We have already discussed the various psychotherapeutic methods used to diminish the pain of childbirth. We have covered the field from as far back as the days of magic and fable to the more recent use of suggestion and hypnosis, the scientific basis of which was demonstrated only after the findings of Pavlov.

It follows that the unfolding of this history shows the strides made from magic to empiricism, and eventually from empiricism to science.

Nevertheless it was the necessity for generalisation and for the mass application of a method of painless childbirth that led the experts to abandon the restricted and specific possibilities of hypnosis and suggestion in favour of a method that not only outstripped the latter but offered a wider spectrum of application to all in any condition.

It was from this very social necessity—for general or mass use—that the concept of psychoprophylaxis was born under the guiding influence of Pavlovian physiology.

This gives to the psychoprophylactic method a concept radically different from all those that preceded it. It may have benefited from Pavlov's elucidation of hypnosis and suggestion, but this does not make it the less divorced from them either in its therapeutic field or in its physiological development. It is this new therapeutic application and its physiological foundation which we wish to describe now.

Once more, let it be recalled that the essential features of the various methods of obstetrical analgesia before the days of psychoprophylaxis were:

(*a*) That they looked upon pain as a symptom.

(*b*) That pain was an inescapable accompaniment of delivery.

(*c*) That the means used to diminish the perception of pain was that of numbing sensation. This was specially the case when drugs were used.

No one had questioned the origin of pain in childbirth; or, if the question had been asked, it had been badly worded. The way in which pain was caused was thought to be strictly physical ; that pain should be legitimately present was never disputed. It was simply a useful symptom of childbirth, and all that needed to be done was to attenuate its unpleasantness.

To question the legitimacy of pain in childbirth, and to solve that problem effectively, required a completely new outlook on the physiology of pain. This new attitude came from Pavlov.

In fact, with the accession of the psychoprophylactic method, obstetrical analgesia becomes invested with a totally new quality. The problem no longer concerns the choice of which method to use to dull the senses, or to abolish the sensory perception of an inevitable and unpleasant symptom. The problem is now to elucidate the physiological processes whereby uterine contractions become painful: and once this is elucidated, to recondition these processes so that the contractions become painless. Hand in hand with this must go the idea that uterine contractions are quite separate from uterine pain, an attitude contrary to the classical one which looked upon contraction and pain as synonymous.

We are therefore dealing with two quite distinct phenomena: uterine contraction and pain. These two phenomena, however, can, as the result of some particular upbringing, be linked together to give rise to painful uterine contraction. It is most important for the reader to grasp the physiological processes at the root of this association, as well as those concerned with its development.

Going back to classical physiology, function is closely welded to the organ which produces it, all physiological activities being stamped, once and for all, into various structures—being kept alive by them and dying when they die.

Each physiological phenomenon was looked upon as having a fate of its own or a doomed necessity governed by some ultimate law. This held true for the pain of childbirth, which was looked upon as definitely ingrained in the contractions of the uterus.

In the light of Pavlovian physiology the pain of childbirth is neither necessary nor inevitable; this conclusion is reached not by virtue of some naïve optimism, but because the pathogenesis* of this pain is based on a new conception of physiological processes.

It is true that each function is a dependent of a definite organ, but this organ possesses functional efficiency in so far as it adapts itself to the vital demands made by our body.

This plasticity or constant ability for adaptation is the work of the nervous system. The nervous system, and its most developed part, the brain, is the apparatus which makes it possible for our body to adapt itself incessantly to the ever-changing state of our environment. Pavlovian physiology, in a way, is the physiology of adaptation; that is, of the constant exchanges between the body and its surroundings. Studied from this angle, each physiological process is the result not only of the structures that have evolved it, but just as much of the external conditions that have induced it. It follows that the presence of such a process is not solely due to a strictly biological need, but depends as well on the human environment.

* Pathogenesis: the development of a disease.

This is the very explanation of the pain of childbirth. It is a mixture of social environment and physiology, and it is as such that it must be approached and solved. The historical events that associated pain with childbirth must be understood and, more so, the way in which it has become ingrained in the brain of women.

From this analysis it will be shown conclusively that pain is linked with the way in which a woman *understands* and *practises* her labour. It corresponds to an individual organisation of the functions of her brain.

This individual organisation can be favourably altered by offering to the woman a new understanding of her labour, coupled with a new way of practising it. It is by a method of education and apprenticeship that this reorganisation of cerebral function in the pregnant woman can be achieved.

In fact, this re-education, based on an appreciation of the pathogenesis of the pain of childbirth, constitutes a *prophylaxis* of that pain. So the psychoprophylactic method, by its rehearsals, amounts to an apprenticeship of childbirth. By learning to deliver herself of her child, by knowing how to do it, a woman ceases to suffer. One could easily say that it is all very simple and it is only a question of having " thought about it ". But, in reality, to have " thought about it " demanded an absolutely new conception of how pain is initiated.

We shall soon see how Pavlovian physiology is applied to the pain of childbirth and how it leads to the psychoprophylactic method. So the whole matter will appear to us as an apprenticeship founded on the physiological processes that it brings to light. We can therefore say rightly that the psychoprophylactic method is a branch of teaching supported by the pillars of physiology.

CHAPTER I

WHAT IS PAIN?

1. THE PROBLEM OF PAIN: ITS COMPLEXITY AND ITS PATHWAYS

IT is by appreciating the mechanism of pain that we seek to battle with it, not simply by dulling our senses. What is pain after all? It is a form of sensation. But as a sensation, it is distinct by virtue of the emotional echoes that it stirs up. To be hurt is to feel something with distinct characteristics; it is not a sting, it is not cold, it is not touch; though each of these sensations may give rise to pain, as would a sharp sting, or a burn or a blow.

So pain is a definite sensation which all of us have experienced to a greater or lesser degree, and which expresses itself in its own fashion, giving rise in us to external signs— grimace or speech.

But what goes on exactly when we feel pain? There are two points which we can assert. The first is a subjective manifestation and consists of the particular sensation we feel. With this goes, to an equal degree, the reactions we show and its not uncommon accompaniment of a pale or flushed complexion; these constitute the objective manifestation of pain.

But there is more to it than just these. There is a common basis for this subjective manifestation as well as its simultaneous external expression. In fact, this represents the essential point; the common starting point of these two apparently different manifestations has its seat in special mechanisms in the brain and it is these mechanisms that fire off painful signals.

It is now universally accepted that pain is the product of special mechanisms in the brain and that it is expressed in

a dual fashion: subjectively by registering a painful sensation, and objectively by miming and outward expressions.

What about the way in which these higher nervous
activities work? This is the fundamental study we have to
undertake in order to grasp how pain comes into being or
disappears. Pain is born as soon as it is picked up at the
periphery of the body by receptors—a process common to
all forms of sensation. The crux of the matter in differenti-
ating it from other sensations lies in its interpretation or
perception. In fact, the hallmark of a painful sensation belongs to its subjective perception. We must also ask the
question, " What is pain that is not perceived as a painful
sensation? "

We can look into our daily life to find examples of the
wide variation shown by the perception of pain. Thus the
commonplace " toothache ", which is barely felt while one
is actively engaged, may become stabbing if our mind
dwells on it should we be inactive. Or headaches which
some people experience when they are upset, and which
soon vanish when they feel serene again. In a similar but
more special way, there is the soldier who is not aware of
his wounds in the heat of battle, or the mystic who shows
not the slightest trace of pain while he is being tortured.
Still other unusual examples are those of mentally un-
balanced people who appear to be completely immune to
stimuli known to be painful.

On the other hand, some people show evidence of real
pain without any legitimate cause for it being found, and
such people are labelled hypochondriacs when, in fact,
they truthfully experience pain.

All these examples make it the more obvious to us that
pain is a complex phenomenon; and we notice that a new
element has found its way into this complex mesh. This
new element is called the psychological aspect of pain;
and at first sight it would seem that the variable factor is
this psychological facet. In reality we know that this facet

is nothing else but a subjective expression of physiological processes—the agitations of the higher nervous centres. Pain does not have two separate parts—a physical one that may be constant and a psychological part which may vary. Pain is an entity, and this unity of pain is effected by the cerebral machinery. To determine this fact was the purpose of a study of the activities of the higher nervous centres, as designed by Pavlov and his followers.

2. Higher Nervous Activity: Its Action and Its Laws

To understand how the brain works, one must try and picture to oneself the many processes going on in the body. The body is capable of many functions, such as respiration, digestion, circulation, etc.; it can also propel itself, and its sensory organs can interpret general or definite sensations. On top of all this, man, *Homo sapiens*, is endowed with a supplementary faculty which places him highest in the animal scale—this is the faculty of speech and, with it, the faculty of thought.

All these add up to functions and activities that must depend on a well-integrated organ. This highly differentiated organ we call the nervous system.

It is the nervous system that imparts life to all our organs; it makes our heart beat, it creates movement in our limbs, and it makes our skin feel. Without it our eyes would be no more than somewhat improved cameras; our stomach but an inert bag; our arms just a system of leverage without any power.

The nervous system, however, does not only give life to this assembly. The body is already alive by virtue of the substance it is made of. The nervous system does more, it *adapts* the working of our body to the changes in its environment. This is its main role, and it is specifically for the exchanges between the body and its surroundings that this specialised " relations officer " has been evolved. In fact, in inferior structures of the simplicity of the amoeba, it is the organ itself, as a whole, which responds to the stimuli of the external environment, by means of a fundamental property of living matter—irritability.

But, as a living body increases in complexity and its various systems and functions become differentiated, external stimulations become more numerous, more varied and more coloured. Then a mechanism appears which is detailed to receive these stimuli and pass them on by readjusting the functions of organs which it represents. This mechanism is the nervous system.

It follows that the nervous system works in accordance with the dual needs of information and response; this is exactly what we call reflex activity.

Reflex activity is this two-way channel of the nervous system, whereby a fixed stimulus (or exciting agent) gives rise to a certain response.

Reflex activity represents therefore the basic unit in nervous activity, and is at the same time the essential link that establishes equilibrium between the individual and his sphere.

If one considers the countless activities of a living being (especially a human being), one soon realises how rich, precise and pliable this reflex activity must be. For this very reason it must be complex as well.

(A) THE CONDITIONED REFLEX

Pavlov has shown that there are two methods by which equilibrium is established between the organism and its surroundings; that is, two types of reflex activity exist.

Firstly, there is a permanent stable reflex activity, created once and for all. It corresponds to an exciting factor which, remaining always the same in the face of a stable element in the environment, always gives rise to the same response. These are termed *absolute reflexes*, and are not conditioned. Simple examples of such reflexes include the production of saliva when food is introduced into the mouth, or blinking to protect the eyes from a blow. Others are more complex, and when integrated may amount to an instinctive reaction.

These " inborn " reflexes add up to the hereditary capital of an individual. They would be sufficient if the exchanges between a living being and its surroundings always stayed the same; that is, if these surroundings were made up only of stable, constant and lasting elements.

In the same way as such elements are sometimes met with in an environment, it is just as true that there are countless factors which are of a transient and changing nature, and with which a living being can come to terms only through the agency of a system of reflexes which is equally transient and changing.

These reflexes, brought into being by the special conditions prevailing in the being's sphere of activity, are called *conditioned reflexes*. They effect a temporary exchange between a factor in the surroundings and an action in the individual. If one ponders over the great number of actions in a being, one can quickly gauge how infinite in its possibilities conditioned reflex activity must be. Just imagine what a web of reflexes, conditioned or absolute, goes into such a simple daily, almost automatic, act as getting ready to go to work; or the still simpler, almost instinctive act of sitting down to a meal.

So conditioned reflex function must be precise, active and variegated and can only be produced by the most differentiated and elaborate part of our nervous system, namely the brain.

If the manner in which a conditioned reflex is created is grasped, this paves the way towards understanding how the brain functions. Let us take as an example a simple conditioned reflex. A dog salivates if meat is introduced in its mouth; this is an absolute or unconditioned reflex. If the introduction of the meat is preceded by the ringing of a bell, and this process is repeated many times, the dog ends by salivating when the bell is rung on its own and no meat given. So an instinctive or hereditary activity—an inborn activity in an individual—has been initiated by a stimulus totally divorced from the one that originally produced it, and this has been brought about solely by a conditioned reflex. This can be reproduced under any condition, provided there has previously been an association between the indifferent or artificial stimulus and the basic or natural stimulus, in such a way that the indifferent one becomes eventually the excitatory factor—but a conditioned excitatory factor.

It is now easier to see how an individual organism can use a conditioned reflex to adapt itself to the constantly changing atmosphere of its surroundings.

What, in fact, happened inside the brain of the dog? It could be argued that the dog was " thinking " about the meat when it heard the bell go. But is that a plausible explanation? And who can prove that the dog was " thinking " of the meat rather than anything else?

Pavlov has demonstrated that it was more fruitful to understand what changes took place in the brain matter itself than to speculate on what the dog was thinking.

This is what happens:

(1) All the stimuli that impinge on our being are transmitted to the brain, be they from our organs of sensory perception, our skin, our muscles, etc., or from the activities of our internal organs, such as the lungs, heart, stomach, etc. They pass up the various nerves and then through the spinal cord to reach the brain.

(2) When a stimulus reaches the brain, it fires off a focus of activity; that is, a certain group of nerve cells starts to become active. This focus of activity directly stimulates function in the absolute reflexes; thus the dog salivates when meat is placed in its mouth, or turns its head towards the sound when the bell rings. In each case the focus of

activity is a different one: the one belongs to the reflex of salivation, the other to that of orientation. But if two foci of activity are fired off at the same time, and this is repeated many times, a connection becomes established between the two foci. If the repetitions have been frequent enough, a permanent communication results. This link gives rise, within the brain matter, to a channel or a pathway between the two foci in such a way that if one is activated by means of its stimulus (the bell) the other becomes activated too without its stimulus (the meat) being present. One focus then activates the other. Hence, the ringing of the bell by alerting its own reflex will, through the medium of the new pathway, activate the reflex of salivation without any meat being required.

This intercommunication between two foci of activity is a temporary one artificially induced by prevailing circumstances and makes it possible for the animal to adapt itself to these circumstances. This liaison constitutes a conditioned reflex.

(B) THE STEREOTYPED DYNAMIC SYSTEM

It goes without saying that our daily activities are made up of innumerable conditioned reflexes. Even the simplest procedure calls for the use of several such reflexes. Generally speaking, conditioned reflexes act as groups, and such a group of conditioned reflexes working together for a definite purpose constitutes a stereotyped dynamic system; stereotyped because such a series of reflexes grouped to produce the same result always has the same sequence; dynamic, because the series follow the fundamental property of all conditioned reflexes—a constant state of flux.

It has already been said that a conditioned reflex results from a temporary association between two foci excited almost simultaneously. It has also been said that our daily activities originate from the stimulation of such a number of foci, while all the associations that add up to the same activity constitute a stereotyped dynamic set. But our daily activities are not only numerous and complex—they vary; each time we do something different we call forth yet another group of associations.

How is this achieved, since it implies that on each occasion a group of foci is fired off while others die down, or vice versa, indefinitely. This phenomenon gives diversity and variation to our activities and, furthermore, confers some form of privilege to certain activities, enabling them to be the only ones to function while the others are resting.

(C) RECIPROCAL INDUCTION

How do cortical centres manage one moment to be active and the next to be resting? Pavlov has shown that this results from one of the fundamental properties of nervous tissue called induction. Each time a cerebral centre or focus becomes active, the brain matter around it reacts by becoming modified so as to function inversely. Excitation therefore induces inhibition, which allows the excitation to be contained and remain concentrated, and not spread to the rest of the brain. Hence, only the excited focus is active and the refractory area that surrounds it is functionless. Anything that reaches this refractory area is not registered by the brain.

Cerebral matter is so made that each focus of activity gives rise to a refractory zone of equal strength, and the greater the activity the more refractory becomes its surroundings.

This makes it easier for us to explain some of the occurrences of our daily life. It explains why, say in a train, when we are concentrating on our paper we do not hear other people's conversation; or why the schoolboy is undisturbed by the street noise while he is absorbed in arithmetic. The hum of conversation in the one case, the noise from the street in the other, travels to the refractory zone induced by the active focus, and is therefore not recorded by the brain.

Later, when painless childbirth is discussed, this fundamental property of nervous tissue will prove useful.

We are now better equipped to understand how some conditioned reflexes are switched on while others are switched off, and how an association of reflexes forming a stereotyped dynamic system is made alert when it is excited by another reflex activity.

(D) THE SIGNALISING ACTIVITY OF THE HEMISPHERES*

We are aware now of how a conditioned reflex starts, and how the conflict between excitation and inhibition causes the reflex to appear and disappear. We know, too, how an arrangement of conditioned reflexes, called a stereotyped dynamic system, is the factor underlying any given activity. This property of the brain hemispheres to engender conditioned reflexes is called its signalising activity. Going back to the formation of a conditioned reflex, we find a neutral excitatory agent displacing the unconditioned agent and taking over from it to behave now as the *signal* for the unconditioned excitation.

This property of signalisation holds true with respect to all the tissues in our body, and, to demonstrate this, more precise problems have to be propounded.

If the brain can give rise to conditioned reflexes derived from external excitatory sources it can be shown too that the same happens as the result of stimuli arising from the working of internal organs. That is, it can be shown that there exists a system of internal signalisation as well.

If we can demonstrate this, we can understand how signals coming from various organs of the body meet in the brain and become *associated*. In fact, if we can prove that such associations take place, we shall have grasped the effect that external circumstances have on the internal pro-

* The brain is made up of a right and a left half, or hemisphere.

cess, and thereby have elucidated the working of our organs.

But let us go further, since we have seen that in man the power of speech has opened up possibilities of a new character. We shall see that speech can be the basis of more conditioned reflexes and thus act as a specific type of internal signalisation. We shall observe what influence words (and more so thought) have on the working of our internal organs. This influence is achieved by the intermediary of associations between signals tied up with words (regardless of form, spoken or written) and signals tied up with the working of internal organs.

To accomplish all this the existence of a means of internal signalisation must be shown. This is what is termed interoception.

(E) INTEROCEPTION

The old dual concept of Bichat dividing the nervous system into somatic and autonomous parts had long ago been exploded. But the honour still goes to the Pavlovian school for having shown the role played by visceral (or autonomous) sensation in influencing cerebral dynamism, and specially in establishing temporary associations.

That school confirmed the main function of the brain in regulating the working of internal organs and adapting them to the environment of the individual.

Many Soviet physicians, above all Bykov, Airapetianz and Kourtzine, have demonstrated the possibility of creating conditioned reflexes starting from interoceptive signals. Many original experiments have been devised, but only a few examples will be mentioned now.

The introduction of pure water into the stomach does not give rise to any gastric secretion; but if this is preceded by an acid solution that induces secretion, then the subsequent instillation of a neutral liquid will cause secretion. In other words, the stimulus (or signal)caused by a liquid which does not have the chemical effect of acid on the gastric mucosa has now become a conditioned excitatory agent.

In another experiment the ureters* of a dog were brought out through the skin, so that urinary excretion could be investigated. The introduction of 100 cubic centimetres of water into the rectum† led to an increase in urinary secretion, this being mediated through an unconditioned reflex. After this had been repeated several times, the simple introduction of the rubber tubing in the rectum gave rise to an increase in urinary excretion. If this procedure was preceded by the blowing of a trumpet, this blare on its own would, after a few times, increase urinary secretion.

This last experiment shows how an external stimulus (the blare of the trumpet) has now become the signal for a visceral activity.

Later it will be shown how similar conditioned reflexes can equally be made to arise from uterine interoception; and this is just what we find between uterine interoception and signals lit up by words—this being now one of the phenomena responsible for pain in childbirth.

We shall now pass to this concept of the spoken or written word as a specific sign—being the second system of signalisation, or second signalising system.

(F) THE SECOND SYSTEM OF SIGNALISATION

Speech as a form of communication (or signalisation) is the result of very complicated processes. Speech is a definite type of signal—it works both directly and indirectly.

Words are externally expressed through two direct excitatory forms: sound, as in the spoken word, and vision, as in the written word.

In an animal speech is nothing else but a direct excitant.

* Ureters : the two tubes which convey urine from the kidneys to the bladder.
† Rectum : the last portion of the large bowel, just before it opens into the anus or back passage.

The spoken word for an animal is just another sound. When a dog is called by its name, the phonetic consonance of the word, linked with the showing of a lump of sugar, creates an association in the brain of that dog so that it eventually moves forward when it is called. One could just as well call him " mat " or " table " and the result would be the same, provided this neutral stimulus, this simple noise, is associated with an absolute reflex. So in the animal only one system of communication exists—the first system—this depending on direct external or internal stimuli.

In man something totally different comes into effect. A word has a significance of a specific nature.

Ivanov-Smolensky has shown that conditioned reflexes could be built starting from words. For example, a conditioned reflex can be started by the word " lane ". The sound " lane " has phonetics of its own and, as far as hearing goes, acts directly on the first system of communication as it does in the animal. But in man it is not just another sound; it is a sound plus something else—a sense.

A word is a sound that carries a meaning. It is this very meaning which determines the nature of the conditioned reflex it has started. Hence in a child the word " road ", or the word " street " with totally different phonetics, will both give rise to the same conditioned reflex as the word " lane ".

In a dog these synonyms give rise to no action, because words to a dog have no meaning; we say that dogs have no sense of speech.

So in man a word is an *indirect* gesture or signal of reality; by its restricted meaning it takes the place of an object, and by its wider meaning that of all objects of the same generic denomination. Thus the word " seat " covers the meaning of the words " chair ", " armchair " or " settee ", etc.

So a word and its broader meaning stands for the object

itself. The general acceptation of words is the product of the accumulated experience of man throughout his evolution. This is why man reacts to the meaning of a word and not just to the sound of a word. Early in childhood this verbal signal replaces the object, and there results eventually a permanent and constant association between the two systems of signalisation.

Words are the substance as well as the carriers of thought, that " internal tongue " of ours.

So words share in the dynamic processes of the brain, and in their behaviour as signals can become linked to other signals, specially interoceptive ones. It is now easier to see how words—written, spoken, thought—can intervene in conditioned reflexes affecting interoception and thereby influence the latter.

In the light of this general study of Pavlovian physiology we are now aware of the way in which stimuli coming both from the external environment of an individual as well as his internal environment (that is, his internal organs) can meet, strike up associations, break them up and tie them up again in the brain.

To man, his external environment is above all his social circle, with its history and its inconsistencies; and his power of speech—in other words his second system of signalisation—is the mirror which reflects on to his brain this complex outer universe. In his mind, organic processes feel the repercussions that history and society have had on this universe. A study of this will reveal how deeply rooted has been the idea of pain in childbirth.

Before embarking on this study we must go into the general problem of pain from a physiological standpoint.

3. The Problem of Pain in Terms of Pavlovian Physiology

The discoveries of Pavlov have thrown a new light on the problem of pain.

Though the many activities of man are mediated through a network of temporary associations derived from conditioned reflexes and fired off by them, it still happens that no physiological phenomenon escapes the ever-active awareness of the brain. Pain is no exception, and its perception by the brain depends on the interplay between excitation and inhibition—that is, by the process of signalisation.

Finally, the perception of pain is linked to the endless permutations of inborn and conditioned reflexes.

Generally speaking pain is not a sensation that is experienced once and for all, and which remains unaffected by external circumstances. There is not such a thing as a " pure " pain, appearing in an undressed fashion; it is always cloaked by its human environment. We saw earlier how a most " natural " form of pain, like that of a toothache, can alter according to what the individual is doing— that is, according to his cerebral activity. It was kept strongly in check when some other focus of activity was holding the field; but it would take over if left as the dominant stimulus. *Pain therefore is a complex cerebral process made up of many components.* This has been confirmed by the work carried out by the Pavlovian school.

(A) TRANSFORMATION OF CONDITIONED REFLEXES

Since 1912 Erofeeva, working in Pavlov's laboratory, had shown how the brain played a major part in the perception of painful sensations and the way in which these underwent alterations.

Here are Pavlov's words from his *Lectures on the Activity of the Cerebral Hemispheres*, about one of Erofeeva's experiments: " Let us take as an example a nocuous stimulus; say, a strong electric current which, when applied to the skin, wounds and cauterises it. This obviously is the unconditioned stimulus of the reflex of self-preservation. The organism reacts to this by a violent motor response that leads either to the removal of the stimulus or the removal of the animal from it. Nevertheless, even in such a case it is possible to use the stimulus to establish a fresh conditioned reflex.

" A nocuous stimulus has been converted into the conditioned one of an alimentary reflex. There was not the slightest trace of a defence reaction evoked by the application to the skin of an electric current of high intensity. Instead, an alimentary reaction was exhibited. The animal turned to face the direction from which food was being held and stretched out its head, licking its lips and secreting saliva.

" The same result could be obtained in the dog if pricked deep enough to draw blood, or if burnt. . . . We have collected absolutely precise proofs that the objective phenomena normally exhibited by animals subjected to strong nocuous stimuli were not observed, even to the smallest degree, in our experiments. When reflexes had been modified in the manner already described, a nocuous stimulus caused no appreciable difference in the pulse rate or respiration of my dogs. Yet differences would undoubtedly have been prominent had not the nocuous stimulus been linked, beforehand, with the feeding reflex."

Drabovitch tells the story of the well-known British physiologist Sherrington who, watching such an experiment, exclaimed: " Now I understand the psychology of martyrs."

Erofeeva's experiment shows that pain can be abolished through the formation of a conditioned reflex.

Conversely, a neutral stimulus can become the starting point of pain. If the ringing of a bell were coupled with a painful stimulus, the ringing on its own could give rise to the sensation of pain.

Thus in another of Erofeeva's experiments—which proved the converse of the above—the buzzing of the electrical apparatus set in motion a painful process.

In human beings, of course, the basic principle remains the same, but it is exhibited after going through a complex network of phenomena. We mentioned this point already, when we said that man's activities with respect to his environment needed the interplay of cerebral functions termed the second system of signalisation. It must again be stressed that speech—whatever its form or development—can play a determining part in these complex processes giving rise to pain.

These were the interesting conclusions reached by Pchonick, and more recently Rogov, after experiments on human beings. Pchonick, by associating a painful stimulus with a buzzing noise, and then the buzzing noise with gentle warmth, converted this warmth into the signal for pain.

This is a case of secondary conditioned reflex (or reflex of the second order) because gentle warmth has now become the signal for pain through the intermediary of the buzzing noise.

In yet another case, not only has the noise become the signal, but the mention of the word " buzzer " started the pain. This experiment demonstrates the physiological import of a word, as expressed by the second system of signalisation. This influence of words has been known for a long time, but its true nature had never been studied.

Rogov in 1953, working in Bykov's laboratory, devised an experiment that provides still further evidence of the importance of signals of this second system.

He heated the skin of his subject by means of a spiral tube through which warm water flowed. Exact degrees of thermal stimulation could thus be applied, and their vasomotor effects were studied by means of a plethysmograph.* At first a temperature of 43° C. was used as stimulus. This produced, by natural reflex action, a state of

---

* Plethysmograph: apparatus used to measure the variations of blood flow in an organ or limb.

vasodilatation* as well as the subjective feeling of painless warmth. A ringing noise is then used as the conditioned exciting factor and, after some twenty to fifty associations (depending on the subject), this noise ends by producing vasodilatation.

If the experimenter then says, " I am going to ring ", that is, replaces the direct stimulus by the verbal one, the natural or unconditioned vasodilator reflex will be evoked in exactly the same manner.

This is then followed by using water at 65° C. At this temperature a natural vasoconstriction is produced, and this is accompanied by a sensation of heat that is painful. When the subject is told, " I am going to apply gentle warmth ", but in fact heat at 65° C. is applied, instead of getting the usual vasoconstriction, there results vasodilatation while the subjective sensation of painless warmth is enjoyed. Here the verbal stimulus contained in the words " I am going to apply gentle warmth " has proved stronger than the effect of a natural excitatory agent in the form of a thermal stimulus of 65° C.

This experiment deserves to be closely analysed as it illustrates vividly the openings made available by Pavlovian physiology in the elucidation of the problem of pain.

Here we have a very real thermal stimulation by 65° C. of heat (known to be painful) negatived as soon as it is preceded by the verbal assurance of warmth only. More than that, this latter stimulus has the positive effect of giving rise to the objective phenomenon of vasodilatation—proved by plethysmography—as well as the subjective sensation of warmth. How does this happen? Simply because sensation here has been completely determined by a cerebral activity conditioned by the second system of signalisation.

In the first half of the experiment, a thermal-conditioned reflex has been created based on a verbal stimulus—the

* Vasodilatation: dilatation of blood vessels.

words " I am going to ring " replacing the conditioned stimulus caused by ringing. The word " warmth " is associated in our everyday life, directly or indirectly, with a real feeling of thermal comfort. Hence the words " I am going to apply warmth " assumes a predominant influence by virtue of a conditioned reflex of the second order, and will even eliminate the effect of direct stimulation by a temperature of 65° C.

It is at this very level in the brain—the level of activity of the second system of signalisation—that we must look for this unusual phenomenon; that is, a pleasant sensation of warmth where a painful sensation of heat should normally be registered.

(B) FUNCTIONAL ACTIVITY OF THE BRAIN

In addition to acquired associations as such, there is a direct influence exerted by the brain on painful sensations.

If the functions of the hemispheres have become exhausted by overwork, or as the result of some intense emotion, there follows a diminution in the efficiency of the various cerebral processes; this applies to inhibition as well. This means that stimuli of sensory origin will set up foci of activity that are likely to spread with greater ease and so give rise to a new climate in the brain. Hence innocuous stimuli may give rise to pain, and extraneous signals are no longer held in check by inhibition and are allowed to assume a painful visceral character.

4. CONCLUSION : PAIN AS AN ENTITY

It follows, therefore, that pain is neither a simple mechanical process nor a mysterious " psychic " one. It is the product of complex cerebral processes in which excitation and inhibition are mutually inductive; the balance between the intensities of these two phenomena is what determines the " threshold " of painful perception.

Pain is an entity for too long looked upon as made up of two separate parts, a subjective and an objective one. Pain is a *whole*, and this unity of action of painful perception is an essential feature of the problem of pain in childbirth.

CHAPTER II

WHAT IS THE PAIN OF CHILDBIRTH?

1. THE FUNCTIONAL RELATIONSHIP BETWEEN THE CORTEX AND THE GENITAL APPARATUS IN WOMEN

PAIN felt in delivery results from interoceptive excitations originated in the uterus and transmitted to the brain, where they become associated with reflexes conditioned by pain.

Pavlov's pupils demonstrated the existence of this genital interoception, then unknown in classical works.

In 1907 Kchichovsky had noticed that conditioned reflexes in animals were altered by menstruation. Gouberbritz in 1922 confirmed similar findings in dogs during the mating season, while Foursikov and Rosenthal studied changes in conditioned reflexes during pregnancy and lactation.

These various observations suggest that the brain is sensitive to functional changes taking place in genital organs. Such an interchange of actions would imply the presence of nervous pathways between the genital organs and the brain.

It was not until 1930 that the work of Kercheev and Sirovatko enriched this suggestion with precise information. These authors had observed, during surgical operations on women, that such procedures as nipping the cervix of the uterus, or injecting tepid fluid into the uterus, or pulling on the suspensory ligaments of the uterus, altered the threshold of sensory perception and led to changes in the rods of the retina.* These can only be explained on the grounds that the responses observed were initiated,

---

* Retina: the innermost perceptive layer of the eyes. Its superficial sensitive cells have the shapes of rods and cones.

through reflex activity, by impulses coming from the internal genital organs.

In recent years more impressive confirmation of the existence of such nervous pathways was revealed by experiments in which the uterus was perfused. In these experiments the only connections left between the animal and its uterus were nervous ones. If the uterus is then stimulated, the pulse rate, blood pressure and respiration rate of the animal are altered; these changes can only be effected by the interoceptors in the uterus sending their experiences via the brain centres (Lotis, Airapetianz, Gambachidzé).

Starting from such interoceptive experiences of the genital organs, the cortex can build up systems of conditioned reflexes. These become recorded by higher centres and, though such sensations do not fall on consciousness, they none the less contribute their share to the physiological activity of these centres.

In 1949 Lotis, by creating a channel between the skin and the uterine inner lining in a bitch, was able to stimulate directly this lining (or mucosa), and by associating the stimulation with feeding, produced a conditioned reflex whereby irritation of the mucosa only gave rise to salivation.

Airapetianz went even further and demonstrated that the cortex could differentiate between two similar stimuli coming from the uterus. Thus by exciting one of the uterine tubes at a rate of 120 stimulations per minute, a positive alimentary conditioned reflex could be established; this could easily be differentiated by the brain from a negative alimentary reflex induced by a rate of 60 stimulations per minute. Similarly, the brain can differentiate uterine sensation felt by water at a temperature of 8°–12° C. from water at 42°–46° C. Hence we can accept the definite existence of nervous pathways linking the internal genital organs with the higher cerebral centres.

2. THE PAIN OF CHILDBIRTH

Peripheral uterine sensations on reaching the brain are translated into consciousness, this being the way contractions are felt during pregnancy. Such contractions are painless, and yet at some stage in labour they become painful. Why is that? This problem remained unsolved until Velvosky studied it.

There is no doubt that at some stage the contractions increase in strength; but this is not a valid explanation because the very same contractions—in spite of their increased intensity—do not give rise to pain in women who have been prepared by the psychoprophylactic method.

Velvosky and his co-workers have shown that emotions and conditioned reflexes interfered with the contractions to make them painful. As they had found out the nature of the pain of childbirth, they had no difficulty in devising a psychotherapeutic method to abolish it.

Pain and childbirth have for so long been associated in the mind of the human race, and have for so long concurred, that they had become synonymous. The normal uterine contraction so necessary for the active progress of labour is mistaken for pain to such an extent that the word " pain " is taken to mean both. In France, labour wards in many units are often referred to as the " Hall of Pain ". The result is a typical conditioned reflex in which the normal painless contraction has become the signal for the occurrence of pain. The characteristic of this reflex is not that it has been acquired by experience, but above all by " common knowledge "—in other words by the influence of speech.

It has already been seen that a temporary connection between words and nervous centres takes place at the level of the first system of signalisation. If a woman is repeatedly told that pain will follow on the first contractions, these will inevitably become the trigger mechanism for pain.

Since the stability of a conditioned reflex depends on the number of times it is repeated, it is easy to understand what a firm bond is knit between pain and contraction by the hundreds of times this is talked of. To make it worse still, tradition amplifies it, and the real experience of others confirms it. Such is the stuff the brain is made of—a stuff that allows associations to turn a contraction into a pain. The simple emotion of the " fear of pain " adds yet another factor which joins in to heighten the pain. Velvosky feels strongly about this factor.

3. The Fear of Pain

The anticipation of pain—not likely in animals—is a conditioned emotion that education has turned into fear. This is well demonstrated in the following experiment sometimes carried out in Soviet labour wards. A plethysmograph is fixed to the arm of a pregnant woman so as to record the vasomotor reactions that accompany painful sensations. If the arm is then pricked with a needle, a definite plethysmographic tracing is obtained. If on a second occasion only the words " I am going to prick you " are said, these words on their own are sufficient to give rise to a similar tracing.

Furthermore, fear is not simply limited to the dread of the pain of childbirth; it extends very often to a fear of complications, such as tearing of the perineum, the use of forceps, Caesarean section, haemorrhages, etc. And here past experience is vivid and real, since it is not very many years ago that post-partum haemorrhages and puerperal fever were common causes of mortality.

Fear can also be connected with the social circumstances of a person. It is a fact that the addition of a child to a family may be a real source of anxiety when the house is too small or the father's income inadequate. The possibility of a war, with its dreadful consequences, is another justifiable cause for worry; and it is natural for a mother to feel depressed about her child's future when her own is overcast.

So the fear that sometimes accompanies childbirth is not infrequently without reason; but in a good number of cases this fear is without foundation.

In an examination of Soviet women Ploticher found that 68 per cent expressed absurd reasons for their fear, such as being afraid that the child would be a freak or an idiot, or thinking that their heart would not stand the strain, etc.

Nowadays, the fear of the complications of childbirth is still more unfounded, as obstetrics has advanced so much that serious haemorrhages and puerperal fever are the exception rather than the rule.

It must not be forgotten, however, that in the present state of society a woman is often given a subordinate place; she still stands for the " weaker sex ". Long before she carries a child she may have experienced unpleasant sexual emotions. Her sexual education is only too often neglected, and this not without repercussions; thus, if she has been ill-prepared for it, her first period, or her first sexual congress, may leave behind enough mental trauma to burden her pregnancy subsequently.

Most women have but a vague idea of the physiological processes involved in conception and in pregnancy, and know nothing about childbirth.

A lack of knowledge sows the seed of fear and feeds the ground on which it grows, and as a rule one dreads the unknown. A poor education allows a woman to become the prey to hearsay. She has heard someone say that childbirth is a painful affair, commonly followed by terrible complications; and right through pregnancy she is being fed with such stories, not least those from her intimate circle— mother, mother-in-law, etc., expounding their own experiences and laying stress on the inevitability of pain and possible complications.

Literature is not blameless either. Many first-class authors have helped in perpetuating this fatalistic idea of pain by describing distressing deliveries, not to mention countless magazines of inferior standard in which childbirth takes place in some mysterious and dramatic manner, and in one case out of two ends by Caesarean section. Such tittle-tattle on pain develops into powerful stimulants that plough their way into the brain.

The role of history is very considerable as it has fostered this fatalistic attitude for centuries, and it has been reinforced by various religions which have coloured a normal phenomenon with some metaphysical justification. (Let it be said, however, that both the Catholic and Protestant Churches have now given their blessing to the psychoprophylactic method.) So anchored by tradition has been this inevitability of pain, that many obstetricians must have felt that the pain of childbirth had become part of the hereditary prerogative of the human race.

4. OTHER CONDITIONED REFLEXES

The multipara,* with her previous knowledge of childbirth, has collected yet other conditioned reflexes which may increase her pain still more. The signals of these reflexes may be the labour ward itself or the appearance of the obstetrician, etc., and on a subsequent occasion these may initiate pain.

In primigravida it is not unlikely for the pain of menstruation to be the portent of the pain of childbirth, since they have a common background, though of varying intensity; and, according to Salganmik, the pain of menstruation could be the basis of complicated conditioned reflexes.

While labour is progressing, if pain becomes marked there will be a tendency for any unrelated stimulus to be drained into the area of painful perception dominating at

* Multipara: a pregnant woman who has borne a child already, as opposed to the primigravida, who is having her first child.

that time the activity of the brain. Such stimuli will only serve to increase the depth of the prevailing pain.

5. PHYSIOLOGY OF THE PAIN OF CHILDBIRTH

Going back over the various factors that govern the nature of pain, we must accept that behind all these conditioned emotions and reflexes there stands high on the list the influence of cerebral activity, of speech, and of education. Experience as such does not play such a decisive part as verbal associations, since pain in the multiparous woman is as great as in the primiparous, in spite of her fuller knowledge of the facts.

On the physiological plane we know that verbal associations work through the first system of signalisation; to that same system will converge conditioned reflexes grouped as dynamic stereotyped units, while it is by means of conditioned connections that painless impulses become painful. This is facilitated still more by exhaustion of the higher centres. On this score, the fear of pain alone is enough to wear out cerebral processes. Thus a sudden upset may make us aware of visceral functions of which we are not normally conscious—giving rise to gastric spasm or to intestinal colic. By electroencephalography* Iakovlev observed interference in the dynamic activities of the brain during pregnancy in the same way that the plethysmograph showed the influence that nervous impulses had on the dynamic activity of the vascular system.

Remembering that the threshold of pain in childbirth will depend on the functional state of the brain, on the conditioned reflexes formed by education, and on the emotional blows inflicted by words, we can now proceed to reorganise the activities of the mind. The psychoprophylactic method will show us the way.

* E.E.G.: the graphic recording of electrical currents developed in the cortex by the various activities of the brain.

CHAPTER III

THE SUPPRESSION OF PAIN
BY THE PSYCHOPROPHYLACTIC
METHOD

THE psychoprophylactic method plans to abolish pain by basing its principles on a knowledge of the genesis of that pain, or, to be more precise, by preventing its occurrence and development in the light of this genesis. The latter is tied up with the special properties acquired by the perception of uterine interoceptive reflexes.

An understanding of the fundamentals of psychoprophylaxis will, therefore, depend on an appreciation of the nervous processes going on in the brain, since these need to be reorganised.

Uterine interoception will impinge on consciousness by creating a focus of excitation, initiated by a painful conditioned reflex. The strength of this focus of excitation, its ability to spread (its irradiation), its creation of persistent painful foci—all these various factors join to contribute to the pain associated with uterine contraction.

Or to express it in a different way, there are two factors involved: the presence of conditioned connections with pain centres on the one hand, and the lack of reciprocal inhibition of these centres on the other. These two sets of phenomena are precisely what psychoprophylaxis sets out to annul, by destroying the obnoxious conditioned associations as well as increasing inhibition to a level high enough to hold back the intrusion of painful stimuli.

These are the essential physiological requirements of the psychoprophylactic method.

1. THE SUPPRESSION OF PAINFUL CONDITIONED REFLEXES

How are reflexes, long conditioned and ingrained in the minds of women, going to be obliterated? They were formed through the help of the second system of signalisation as the results of stories dramatising childbirth and giving it a background of agony. This has amounted to a negative education propagating the belief in painful contractions arising from uterine interoception.

In order to destroy this belief, it is necessary to destroy prejudices based on ignorance. Hence, one of the objects of the method is to enlighten the woman by instructing her about the phenomena involved in childbirth, the purpose being to convert delivery from the idea of pain to a series of understood processes in which uterine contraction is the leading phenomenon.

Uterine contraction then becomes a simple and obvious physiological process which is responsible for the dilatation of the cervix in the first stage of labour and for the delivery of the foetus in the second stage. Labour thereby leaves the high-lights of phantasmagoria for the quiet shadow of physiological reality.

This *undramatising* of labour is the first step towards destroying any distressing associations. Furthermore, by removing apprehension, fear and depressing thoughts, it raises the threshold of cortical activity and thereby the level of the basic processes of excitation and inhibition. These play no inconsiderable part in the long run.

The second step consists of the formation of new conditioned reflexes. Here, if uterine stimuli are associated long enough with sufficiently strong stimuli elsewhere, a conditioned reflex may result, linking the two foci of activity set up by the respective stimuli. The nervous connection between these two foci takes place at the level of the second system of signalisation, and is brought about by the special apprenticeship of the future mother.

During the preparatory stages of pregnancy this connection is effected by giving practical lessons corroborating
uterine contraction with delivery.

Along what lines should these lessons run?

They should aim at teaching things of definite use during
delivery for two main reasons:

1. Because by demonstrating use, the necessity of the
   apprenticeship is made more impressive.
2. Because in labour there are mechanical and biological
   components that cannot be underestimated.

These two aims can be fulfilled by teaching breathing
exercises of a *specific nature*.

Normal respiration works by an inborn reflex. By modi-
fying the rhythm of breathing, a conditioned reflex is
initiated as a sort of " branch " of the normal reflex. The
repeated teaching of this new respiratory style leads to the
formation of a new conditioned reflex, which we may call
the contraction-respiration reflex.

Uterine contraction, as a sequel of this, becomes the
signal for a specific respiration and not any longer for pain.
In other words, as soon as uterine contractions appear the
conditioned reflex channels the stimuli from the uterine
interoceptors into the new centre of respiratory rhythm for
the latter's own benefit. This diversion away from foci of
pain represents an analgesic manoeuvre.

The exercises taught should be of *shallow and quick*
breaths. These are *useful* exercises, not only because they
have created a conditioned association, but because they
have a useful biological purpose. They help oxygenation of
the blood, and bring about a favourable mechanical relationship between diaphragm* and uterus.

So in the first stage of labour, while the cervix dilates,
this *positive manoeuvre* is practised by the parturient; similarly, in the second stage the previous teaching of *controlled*

* Diaphragm: the muscular separation between chest and abdomen.

expulsion will enhance the practical efforts of uterine contraction. This is the method by which the old belief in pain is recanted *at the same time* that new associations are welded together for a useful purpose.

2. STRENGTHENING INHIBITION

Psychoprophylaxis, as mentioned before, has two objects. The first is to remove any detrimental focus, and the second to limit the spread and duration of painful cerebral excitation transmitted by the uterine interoceptors. It has also been shown that this spread depends on the phenomenon of irradiation controlled by the antagonistic effect of inhibition.

When a woman is taught a useful manoeuvre, should this lead to the formation of a new conditioned association, there follows a corollary in the nature of a strengthening of this much-needed inhibition.

In fact this new conditioned association is nothing else but the summation of two foci of activity (the first depending on uterine interoception and the second on the woman's preparatory training) to form a new focus. This focus induces around it, during excitation, large zones of inhibition that limit the diffusion of activity. Meanwhile, the activity of this focus is being reinforced by the interest the woman shows in her pregnancy and in the progress of her labour as a result of the lectures she has previously attended.

All this put together—the knowledge of biological processes and the rehearsing of useful manoeuvres—not only reshapes cerebral attitude as already shown, but increases the potential energies of the various foci, and with it the efficiency of labour.

CHAPTER IV

THE PHYSIOLOGICAL VALUE OF READ'S METHOD

BY the time that the experiences of thousands of women had proved beyond doubt the possibility of childbirth without pain, incredulity gave place to a scepticism based on misunderstanding. It was held by some that the " so-called " childbirth without pain did not in fact " do away " with pain, but simply reduced pain considerably by alleviating the fears, anxieties and apprehension previously associated with childbirth. This method, by unburdening the woman of the weight of culture and civilisation, gave her an easier delivery. She had, so to speak, returned to the unadulterated primitive state. Hence the use of phrases like " childbirth without fear ", or " childbirth without apprehension ", or " natural childbirth ". The psychoprophylactic approach happened to be one of the many, the very many ways, of achieving this.

Perhaps the most widespread method of " natural " childbirth is the one elaborated by Grantly Dick-Read. But if his principles and techniques are briefly analysed, it will be seen without difficulty how different they are from those of psychoprophylaxis.

Read misses completely the fundamental principle of the conditioned reflex, the importance of the indissociable part played by a signal, and the biological value of words as a second system of recording reality. Read has therefore remained impervious to the intricacies and role of consciousness. He has failed to realise that consciousness is part and parcel of higher nervous activity and that it depends on organic nervous pathways. He has not been aware of the fact that the " contents " of the mind are the results of marks left by verbal symbols, and therefore represent in the brain the image of ideas perpetuated in one's environment by history, culture, philosophy, etc. He has turned his back on this fundamental point in the abolition of pain, namely the powerful and immediate effect of the mind on biological phenomena.

Read explains the pain of childbirth in a different way. Uterine contraction produces stimuli that reach the brain, already perverted by social influences. The brain gives a " false interpretation " to these stimuli, mistaking them for painful ones. This misinterpretation, reinforced by the fear that besets the woman during delivery, fires off a defence mechanism which is governed by the sympathetic system. This defence mechanism expresses itself essentially by a uterine contraction, chiefly by that of the circular muscular fibres of the neck of the uterus. The result is a tendency for the cervix not to dilate, and therefore stand in the way of the work done by the longitudinal muscular fibres of the uterus. From this conflict springs " true " pain. This is the essence of the theoretical belief of British psychosomatic practitioners. It consists in reassuring the woman so as to reduce fear, in numbing her consciousness so as to decrease the pernicious influences of society, and in encouraging her to relax so as to offset the main feature of the defence mechanism.

Reassuring a woman is a way of giving her confidence in her labour and her obstetrician. Read has achieved this effectively by rational and educational means. But he has, above all, created in his subjects a state of ecstasy, a mystic impulse to go back to this primitive pureness. The subjects shared with him this mystic exaltation, which is far from being one of the least important facets of his method.

The dulling of consciousness amounts to giving the woman a second place; the idea seems to be to induce in her a pleasant torpor, some sort of a day-dream as in the slumber of sunbathing. Any tendency to formulate organised thought must be deliberately repressed and turned into a fanciful dream.

Muscular contraction is abolished by relaxation; Read, therefore, insists that relaxation should be one of the supporting pillars of his method.

If we analyse Read's method in the light of Pavlovian physiology, we find it easy to understand why he has been only partially successful.

Normally, a complete state of relaxation will lead to a diffuse inhibition of the cortex. A conditioning of this relaxation will result in the cortical inhibition that precedes sleep. But muscular relaxation can also be the result of the inhibition reciprocally induced by a cortical centre of intense activity. This type of inhibition is much superior to the one that prevails just before sleep. This powerful cortical excitation is precisely what Read creates by the mystic exaltation associated with labour in general, and uterine contraction in particular. Its sequel is the diversion and absorption of painful conditioned reflexes, as well as the blocking of stimuli from outside or from unfavourable muscular activity.

Read's method, in fact, contains two contradictory principles. The mystic exaltation is a positive influence, while relaxation is a negative one. According to which of the two has the greater effect, success is more or less obtained; but it is never as complete as Read indicates.

Read's method (and more so all the derivatives that are being elaborated at the moment) does not aim at abolishing pain as such, but rather the physiological climate that worsens pain—a climate darkened by fear and anxiety. The appellation of " childbirth without pain " would be a misnomer for such methods.

Read did not seek to abolish pain directly, as he had not attempted to discover its actual mechanism. Unfortunately, ever since Read started his method, the practice of " natural " childbirth has become poorer. Its positive factor made up of a half-mystical and half-rational mixture, has completely disappeared. In many ways the mystic influence that Read had on his patients is not easy to copy, as it depends undoubtedly on the personality of the obstetrician. But this is not the main point; the real difficulty is met with at the level of reasoning, due to the fact that only a limited proportion of women are likely to yield to his mystification asking them to go back to the pureness of a primitive state, to " decivilise " themselves in a way. The others, on the contrary, would rather be reasonably informed.

There was no better field conducive to the growth of a pseudo-science than the one offered by a theory of muscular contraction; and Read has grafted this willy-nilly on the empirical practice of his art, sacrificing meanwhile some physiological truths.

This doctrine of natural childbirth is fast becoming a simple matter of muscle activity, like some stupid athletic performance carried out without rhyme or reason. Those who thought they had applied Read's method by training muscular activity, and were surprised at the poor results they obtained, were not aware that what they had left out was the mystical element that gives to Read so much ascendancy.

We do not wish to condemn the benefit that the rational physical education of a pregnant woman confers on organic functions—as it would do in anybody else. But this is not the same as childbirth without pain. Besides, accomplished athletes are no better off than their sedentary fellow-women when it comes to the pain of delivery.

" Painless childbirth " is founded on its effect on the brain, a brain that organises the activities of the body and is always in touch with the functions of its organs. It is by reshaping nervous function, and the influence of consciousness, that one teaches a woman to deliver herself without pain.

PART III
LECTURES

INTRODUCTORY LECTURE: PREGNANCY

THE training of patients is not the work of one person only. It is the work of a team which, in spite of its many demonstrators, does safeguard the uniformity of the method.

Each member of the team plays an active part in the training, this being a very important point in enriching the joint efforts of the team and thereby guaranteeing the success of the practice.

There can be no dissociation between the training of the subject and the care she will be given in the labour ward. The only way to make certain of this is for each member of the team to work on both units. We have found that this paid us dividends by improving our results.

We thought it wise to make each lecture as personal as possible. We have therefore done our best to make them " live " by bringing into them the personalities of the various members of the team, so as to create diversity.

The various lectures are given, in the order they are printed, during the last two months of pregnancy, with the exception of this introductory lecture, which is given during the third month.

PROCESSES TAKING PLACE DURING PREGNANCY

The psychoprophylactic method requires that during a woman's preparation for a painless delivery she should be taught as succinctly as possible the physiology of pregnancy. This teaching can then be followed by a study of the minute details of the mechanism of delivery.

Most women—and let us be frank about this—have but a limited knowledge of the various stages of pregnancy. As far as the anatomy of their genital organs goes they know they have a uterus and two ovaries, but here again they place these ovaries at changing levels as circumstances may require! As far as physiology goes, our future parturients have but a superficial and simple conception of the working of their organs; so it is not strange for them to find it difficult to understand impregnation, not to mention childbirth.

(A) ANATOMY

It is not enough to study the various organs that make up the genital tract as isolated structures. These must be seen in their right perspective in the *pelvis*; that is, the re-

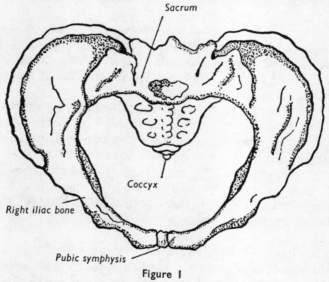

Figure I

lationship of sexual organs to the other contents of that pelvis must be studied.

What exactly is the pelvis? It is in the nature of a shell, of a bony envelope formed almost entirely by two bones. These are the iliac bones, which we may well call the hip bones.

These bones, to which are hinged the lower limbs, are

not welded to each other. If a finger is run along the upper border, or iliac crest, of one of these bones, from back to front, one notices that they articulate with each other across the mid-line in front by a *symphysis*. This, called the pubic symphysis, is a bridge of tissue holding the two bones together.

At the back these hip bones articulate with the vertebral column (or backbone) short of its lowermost part, which is made up of the sacrum and coccyx.

This arrangement of bones forms a real osseous belt,

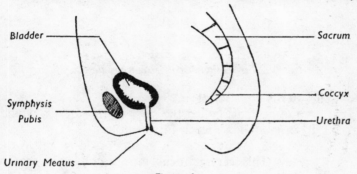

Figure la
Cross-section of pelvis showing bladder

shaped like a funnel with its wide part facing upwards. Within this cavity are sheltered many organs. Which are they?

At the front, almost flush against the pubic symphysis, lies the bladder. The bladder communicates with the outside by means of a tube called the urethra, the opening of which is called the urinary meatus.

Behind the bladder sits the uterus or womb. The uterus is a muscle, that is, an organ possessing the inherent and essential power to contract. This muscle in its ordinary (non-pregnant) state feels firm to the finger, but during pregnancy it undergoes a marked softening. There is no need to describe the ways in which the muscle is arranged, but it must be remembered that the womb is a hollow muscle, that is, a muscle with a cavity in it—the uterine cavity.

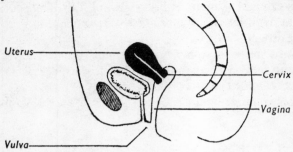

Figure 1b
Cross-section of pelvis showing uterus

The uterus consists of:
1. An upper part called the *body* of the uterus, which, like the bladder, has a forward tilt.
2. A lower part or neck, an inch or so long, called the *cervix*. This cervix opens into a collapsible cavity called the *vagina* (or front passage). This in turn opens to the outside via the *vulva*.
3. Between those two parts of the uterus there is an intermediate narrow portion like a waist.

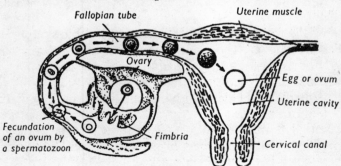

Figure 2

Behind the uterus lies the terminal part of the large bowel, that is, the *rectum*. It opens externally through the *anus* (or back passage).

So the uterus is in a definite position facing the bladder at the front and the rectum at the back. This position suggests already the cause of the urinary and intestinal symptoms so frequent in pregnancy.

Examining the genital apparatus more closely, we see that the uterus does not just sit in the pelvic cavity. Quite the contrary. It hangs from the bony sides of the pelvis by

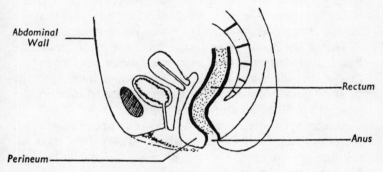

Figure 2a

Cross-section of pelvis showing rectum

means of three pairs of straps or ligaments (the round ligaments in front, the utero-sacral ligaments at the back, and the broad ligaments at the sides). These ligaments allow the uterus a fair degree of freedom of movement.

On each side of the uterus are situated the *ovaries* (Figure 2). Each ovary contains *ova,** these ova having been there since birth.

Each ovary is connected to the uterine cavity via a tube which is a prolongation of the body of the uterus, and which is termed a *Fallopian tube* (Figure 2). This tube varies in length from four to six inches. Like the uterus this tube

* Ova: the plural of the Latin word *ovum*, meaning an egg.

has muscular properties. At its end, furthest from the uterus, this tube expands funnel-wise to embrace the ovary. This splayed-out opening is called the *ampulla* and its edges are fringed and festooned to form the *fimbria*. Finally, the inside of the Fallopian tube is carpeted with fine hair-like processes, or *cilia*, which will be mentioned again later.

(B) PHYSIOLOGY

We shall try to make this as simple as possible, though paying special attention to the part played by the ovary.

Without fear of making a mistake, it can be said that the only, but complex, role of the ovary is *reproduction*.

The ovary participates in the mechanism of menstruation in its role as an organ of *internal secretion*. This means that it manufactures hormones and pours them into the body. These hormones are of great importance in the general sexual behaviour of the woman.

Similarly, the ovary fulfils its role as an organ of *external* secretion. Regularly—once in about twenty-eight days—it releases eggs or ova. Finally, after an ovum has become fertilised, the ovary, by means of its hormonal secretions, nurtures the ovum on the uterine bed.

The ovary is a " pile of ova ". It has been roughly compared to a bunch of grapes, each seed being an ovum. It is generally accepted that both ovaries do not function simultaneously every month, but in turn and roughly alternately. Each month, at a definite time, the functioning ovary releases an ovum. This phenomenon of the shedding of an ovum is called *ovulation*.

A great deal of research has shown that ovulation takes place about the fourteenth day of the cycle in a woman with a regular menstrual cycle of twenty-eight to thirty days. If one had to be more precise, one would say that ovulation takes place between the twelfth and the fifteenth day. This, however, is not an absolute rule; and in any one person it

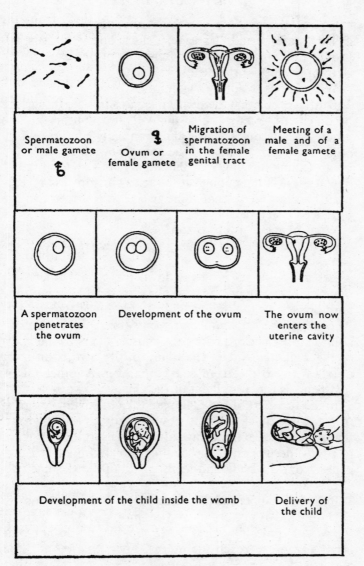

Figure 3

can be a few days late or a few days early. Hence the so-called " safe period " is a very short one, and lasts approximately from the twenty-third day of one cycle to the sixth or seventh of the next.

What happens during ovulation?

During each cycle the ovary increases in size. Its surface becomes congested, and a small fissure appears at one point. This becomes bigger and eventually ruptures, liberating an ovum. Normally, the ovary cannot be easily felt by an examining finger in the vagina; but at the time of ovulation it is big enough to be felt. This process repeats itself every cycle, so that some twelve to fourteen ova are produced every year.

What happens to this ovum?

Its future will differ depending on whether or not it becomes fertilised.

Let us follow its progress down the genital tract. The ovum is first caught by the fimbria of the Fallopian tube and directed to the uterus. This migration of the ovum is dictated by the *peristaltic movements* (muscular propulsive contractions) performed by the muscle fibres in the walls of the Fallopian tube. The ovum on its own is an inert object with no means of self-propulsion. Another factor that helps is the movement of the cilia.

In the first part of the Fallopian tube the ovum gets propelled fairly quickly but it slows rapidly lower down, so that it takes some three days after ovulation for the ovum to reach the uterus. If the ovum is not fertilised, it is expelled from the body and menstruation follows some two weeks later.

But what happens if the ovum meets a spermatozoon?

Unlike the ova, spermatozoa are motile and move about the way tadpoles do. They move rapidly and do not wait for the ovum to reach the uterus. They " nose out " the ovum and make for it—being attracted to it—so that within two to three hours sperms have reached the Fal-

lopian tube. It is within the latter that the spermatozoon
(or male element) meets the ovum (or female element), and
their union gives rise to *fertilisation*.

There are some eighty to one hundred and fifty million
spermatozoa for each cubic centimetre of spermatic fluid,
yet only one will fuse with the ovum to fertilise it.

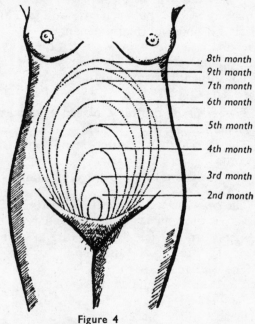

8th month
9th month
7th month
6th month
5th month
4th month
3rd month
2nd month

Figure 4
Height of fundus during pregnancy

This egg will undergo remarkable changes on its three
to five days' trip to the uterus. When it gets there its
wandering life is over, as it becomes attached or fixes itself
to the lining of the uterus. It then burrows its way into that
lining, embedding itself. This is called the *implantation* of
the egg.

The first stage of gestation (or pregnancy)—as already
seen—is the result of co-ordination between the nervous

system and the ovarian hormonal secretions in such a manner that the uterine lining is ready for implantation. At the same time the rest of the body undergoes several changes.

As a rule implantation takes place in the fundus of the uterus, on its back or posterior wall. (Occasionally, however, it may occur in atypical places like the fimbria, the Fallopian tube, etc., but such cases are rare and need not be discussed under normal pregnancy.)

After more development we reach that stage in the life of an ovum at which it has become a mature egg. A study of its constituent parts is helpful.

It is made up of:

1. The *embryo*, centrally placed and surrounded by *amniotic fluid*.
2. The *placenta* (the " after-birth ") and the umbilical cord.
3. The *membranes*—being three in number.

1. The *embryo* soon becomes the foetus and is endowed with active movements right through pregnancy. These movements are first felt by the future mother somewhere between the fifteenth and the twentieth week.

2. The *placenta* is a sort of fleshy " cake-like " mass bound to the wall of the uterus on one surface and linked with the foetus, via the umbilical cord, on the other. These two surfaces of the placenta are quite distinct. The foetal surface (carrying the cord) is smooth and blue in appearance. The uterine side is red and has an uneven surface crossed by furrows dividing it into *cotyledons*.

The placenta directs exchanges between mother and foetus. In fact, the vessels from the foetus run through the cord reaching the placenta, where they break to form the *villi* that are bathed in maternal blood. This blood in turn reaches the placenta from the uterine arteries that ramify in the uterine muscle to form real pools of blood.

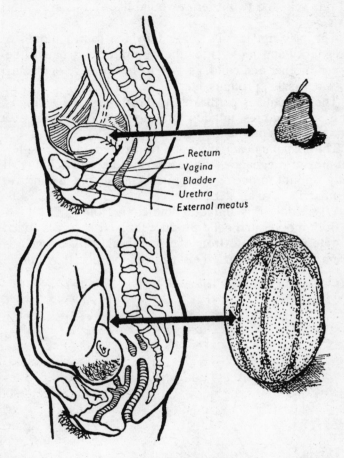

Rectum
Vagina
Bladder
Urethra
External meatus

Figure 5
Comparative development of the uterus

The *umbilical cord* is some 20 inches long, and consists of one vein and two arteries wound like spirals around its axis.

The placenta is fully formed by the fourth month of pregnancy and looks after the respiratory exchanges between mother and child, as well as the nutritive ones, such as water, salts, proteins, etc.

The placenta is permeable to hormones and vitamins, and manufactures, in addition, hormones of its own with known effects on the uterus, ovaries, etc.

The *amniotic fluid* is clear and transparent in the first few months of pregnancy, but near term it becomes cloudy. It may amount to one or two pints, being simple in constitution, and above all sterile.

Where does this amniotic fluid come from?

Both mother and child produce it. To it becomes added a watery transudate from the umbilical cord, as well as urine from the foetus. This will remind one that during

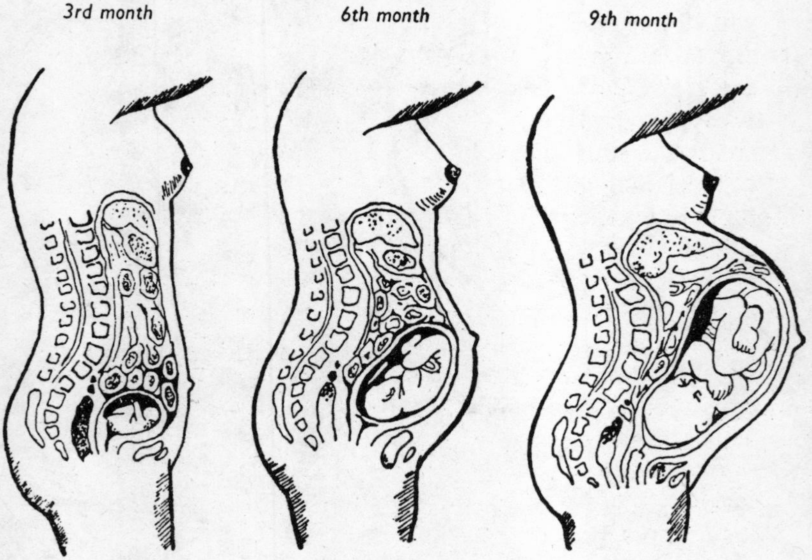

3rd month   6th month   9th month

Figure 6

pregnancy—and especially from the fifth month onwards —all the organs of the foetus are formed. They have a limited function, but they function just the same. This holds true for the liver, kidneys, bladder, bowels, etc., but *not* the lungs.

This amniotic fluid is being continually ingested by the foetus and exerts a protective action on it, not only as a shock absorber during pregnancy but also during delivery.

3. The *membranes* ensheath the egg, thus creating a cavity or " chamber " that is completely waterproof and sterile.

Let us now study the evolution of that egg from implantation to delivery.

During the first two months the fertilised ovum is said to be in its *cystic stage*. It is then no more than a spherical object covered with fine root-like projections called *villi*. By the end of this stage it measures $1\frac{1}{2}$ to 2 inches.

The next stage—from the third month—is called the *embryonic* stage. Some villi disappear during that period, while others become part of the placenta. In spite of an increase in size, the embryo has not yet filled the uterine cavity completely, and now measures from 3 to 4 inches.

By the sixteenth or seventeenth week its size has increased to some 6 to 8 inches. That period of pregnancy is of special interest to the future mother, because it is around those dates that she first becomes aware of movements inside the uterus.

The embryo has now passed into the *foetal stage*—from about the fifth month. It is slowly taking on all the characteristics of the future child. During that stage another important sign appears. It is the presence of viscous or glairy matter blocking the opening in the cervix. This is called the *mucous plug*.

At seven months the foetus measures about 16 inches, reaching the size of 20 inches as delivery nears, and weighing about seven pounds.

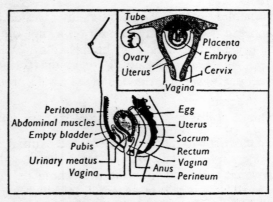

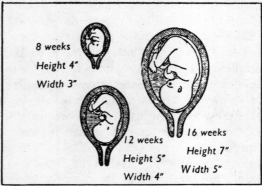

Figure 7a

So much for these anatomical and physiological sketches of the genital organs. Outside this sphere proper, other changes are taking place, and these should be briefly reviewed.

THE ABDOMINAL WALL

As the size of the uterus increases, the abdominal wall assumes, from the fourth month onwards, a typical curvature, while the muscles forming the " abdominal belt " tend to become slack. In addition, a vertical dark line appears in the mid-line. It is first noticed during the fifth to sixth month, and is most prominent above the umbilicus (navel).

THE BREASTS

Here changes take place early in pregnancy. They consist briefly of an enlargement of the breasts with a sensation of pins and needles and of pigmentation (or darkening) of the nipples. The nipples show as well little elevations called the tubercles of Montgomery, these being accessory mammary glands.

Throughout pregnancy the whole body undergoes slow and progressive alterations, and these will demand certain necessary hygienic precautions.

THE HYGIENE OF PREGNANCY

If we still have to be persuaded that reasonable hygiene during pregnancy exerts a favourable effect on mother and child, we can refer to the experimental work of Professor Fodiajina. His work has shown that the intra-uterine development of the foetus depends on its environment. This, in turn, is determined by complex processes taking place in the maternal system. These processes are closely linked with the way the pregnant woman lives.

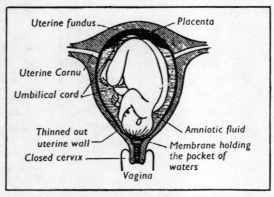

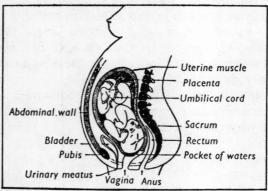

Figure 7b

For purposes of clarity, hygiene during pregnancy will be discussed under the following four headings:

(1) Alimentary hygiene.
(2) Body hygiene.
(3) Mental hygiene.
(4) Medical follow-up.

Before going any further it must be pointed out that childbirth without pain has, by virtue of its psycho-prophylaxis, brought about far-reaching changes in the general hygiene of pregnancy.

Whereas in the past a woman had little knowledge of pregnancy or delivery—and therefore played no more than a passive role—now she is eminently active from start to finish, thanks to an instruction based on science; and we must keep in mind that the atmosphere that surrounds her during her pregnancy will be a determining factor in the success of her delivery without pain.

(A) ALIMENTARY HYGIENE

Meals should be taken at regular intervals, and should be thoroughly chewed. The food allowance during pregnancy should be slightly higher than normal, but must not be excessive, as conditions such as dyspepsia or hypertension may result and hinder the welfare of both mother and child.

Nausea, vomiting and loss of appetite are as useless to pregnancy as pain is to delivery, and can be dealt with by taking small frequent meals.

A well-balanced diet should be taken, proteins, fats and carbohydrates being taken in their correct proportion.

The following meals can be recommended: Grilled or roasted meats; roasted chicken; boiled new-laid eggs; fresh sea or river fish, either steamed or fried. Pastries, rice, potatoes, green vegetables—preferably uncooked—and animal and vegetable fats.

Cheeses (with the exception of the fermented variety), fresh or cooked fruit and milk are highly recommended.

Table salt (sodium chloride) should be slightly restricted during the first eight months. A good working rule is to cook with salt, but not to add any before eating. During the last month it is wise to use salt sparingly. The question of a low salt diet is, however, best left to the obstetrician-in-charge.

There are other minerals that are essential for the proper development of the foetus, and these include iron, iodine, phosphorus and calcium, all of which are provided by a well-balanced diet.

Meals to be condemned include highly spiced ones, game, salted meats, preserves, wines with a high alcoholic content, alcohol, liqueurs and aperitifs.

Take wine and coffee in moderation. Water is the best drink there is.

Vitamins. These chemical substances, circulating in the maternal system, contribute to the proper development of the foetus and to its delivery.

Vitamin A governs the functioning of mucous membranes and is to be found in milk, salt-water fish and butter.

Vitamin B is of importance in the proper assimilation of food in the intestinal tract. A deficiency of this vitamin gives rise to neuritis. It is present in milk, rice, greens, mushrooms, chicken and eggs.

Vitamin C is a constituent of oxidation processes in the body. It is essential to the proper formation of bone marrow, and strengthens the toughness of blood vessels and red blood cells, but is destroyed by the overcooking of food.

A deficiency of this vitamin decreases body resistance to infection, and may lead to renal damage and bleeding from the gums.

It is found in fresh potatoes, tomatoes, lemons and oranges.

Vitamin D helps the body to absorb calcium; large amounts should not be taken as it tends to increase the weight of the child unnecessarily. Here again the doctor's advice should be sought when additional amounts are required in twin pregnancies or during very cold weather.

Milk, eggs and cocoa are rich in vitamin D.

Vitamin E plays a part in furthering the multiplication of cells in the embryo. It has been called the anti-abortive vitamin, as it enhances a healthy development of the ovum at the start of gestation. Cereals, milk, butter and egg yolk contain it.

Vitamin K. This is the anti-haemorrhagic vitamin. It is found in green vegetables, tomatoes, cauliflower, spinach and fresh fruits.

All these vitamins are obtainable as medical preparations, and can be prescribed by the practitioner if he thinks fit.

(B) BODY HYGIENE

Garments and underwear. It is advisable that they should be sufficiently loose to fit all the stages of pregnancy, and be in no way so tight as to hinder the circulation of blood. They should at the same time afford sufficient protection against cold.

Brassières should have deep enough supports, so as to hold the breasts well up and close to each other.

Footwear should follow the same personal pattern as that previously acquired.

Often women ask about a pregnancy belt, which they want to wear from the third month onwards. What it is supposed to hold is difficult to see, and it should not be advised. There are, however, a few exceptions, as in a weakness of the anterior abdominal wall following an operation, or from the muscular atrophy of poliomyelitis. In such cases there exists a medical indication for wearing them.

We would rather see this passive attitude of wearing a belt replaced by the *active* attitude of physical culture, whereby the abdominal muscles will forge their own belt. This is the ideal state of affairs, as an act which meets the demands of pregnancy makes at the same time for better delivery. Furthermore, it benefits feminine contours after childbirth.

Toilet. This should not differ from the normal routine before pregnancy. Baths are taken as usual.

The external genitalia should be given frequent attention, and on no account should douching be practised unless prescribed by a medical man—and only by a medical man.

During the first five months the pregnant woman should limit her activities during those days of the month that would normally have corresponded to her periods. Long journeys and carrying of heavy things over the arm should be restricted during such days.

Sexual congress. Unless forbidden for medical reasons, there is no taboo during pregnancy except during the last month, when total abstinence is the rule.

Physical activities. These remain the same as before pregnancy. Sedentary people will benefit from an hour's walk, without finding it tiring.

Those who are used to sports will find it advantageous to indulge in them, provided they are not violent. Swimming is highly recommended, provided it is not overdone.

All modes of travel are safe during pregnancy, be it by train, ship, aeroplane, underground, bus or bicycle.

Towards the end of pregnancy there is a tendency for the blood return from the legs to be impaired. It is wise to sleep with the legs slightly raised, and not to stand for too long.

(C) MENTAL HYGIENE

Experience has shown that the enacting of labour reflects, in most cases, the climate that has prevailed during pregnancy. Hence the importance of the attitude assumed by the pregnant woman towards these recent, but normal, changes in her own body.

On no account must she adopt a passive attitude during that period. Only a constant, firm and resolute adaptation (resulting from her knowledge of the laws of nature in pregnancy and childbirth) can reward the mother's efforts by crowning her pregnancy with a child born not only without pain, but in the midst of joy.

This knowledge of obstetric physiology is acquired by the young patients during antenatal lectures, which are constantly enriching and correcting ideas which they had already formulated on the subject. Unfortunately, the majority of these ideas are not often correct; they have been neither brought up to date nor completed in educational programmes.

This antenatal course of lectures would be easier and more efficacious had husband and wife received, in good time, a scientific education relating to the processes that have governed the main transformations in their bodies. Such a prepubertal education no more exists than does a comprehensive prenuptial one.

The true facts that are revealed and demonstrated during this antenatal course collide with erroneous ideas housed in the minds of women—vestiges of the atmosphere in which they have been brought up. Their own environment is, furthermore, a source of difficulties of all sorts, of worry, of anxiety, and of sorrow.

A welcomed and wanted pregnancy, plus a happy conjugal life, are propitious factors of importance. A husband versed in the principles of childbirth without pain will offer his wife active support which can but increase her chances of success. He will see that she keeps regular hours for her meals, goes to bed and gets up regularly; all this taking place in a peaceful atmosphere, without overwork and away from the company of agitated and noisy people. Romantic and journalistic writings should be banned; so should theatrical pieces and films that have dramatic passages centring on pregnancy and childbirth. In the same way one should not listen to people who indiscriminately find delight in spreading erroneous and tragic stories about childbirth. This demands that the future mother should be on the alert all the time.

(D) MEDICAL FOLLOW-UP

Every pregnant woman should be under medical supervision in her own interest as well as that of her child.

The first antenatal attendance takes place about the third month. It will consist of a gynaecological examination; a chest examination (both clinically and by X-rays) to exclude any possibility of tuberculosis; a blood examination to exclude syphilis;* an examination of the heart and of the blood pressure and, finally, a urine examination.

With this first attendance will start the re-education of the future mother. She should be treated with the utmost care by the staff of the ancillary medical departments. The doctor-in-charge will try to get a rough idea of how nervous she is so as to guide her and, if at all necessary, to refer her to a psychotherapist working within the compass of the psychoprophylactic principles of childbirth without pain.

It is most important to start the hunting down of old conditioned associations from the very first contact with the parturient.

Every month the woman attends an antenatal clinic. Her progress is carefully recorded. She has an obstetric

---

* The father should equally be examined. (Blood tests are also done to find the patient's blood group.)

examination, her blood pressure is taken, urine is tested, and she is weighed. She should gain not much more than two pounds every month. The obstetrician will repeat the most important rules of hygiene; he will see that she sleeps well, and will forestall any tendency to constipation.

When questions are asked during such consultations the doctor should answer in a tone of voice that is informative, so as to reinforce all new conditioned associations. Special problems like unmarried motherhood, etc., are dealt with by almoners, who help the woman solve her problem as well as possible.

Let us close by underlining the point that the preparation proper, the organised prenatal examination, the ever-warm welcome given to the future mothers by the administrative staff, must all work towards the same end; namely, creating for the mothers a psychohygienic atmosphere that will help them to unshackle the old associations and give birth to perfectly healthy children.

THE PAIN OF CHILDBIRTH: HOW AND WHY
IT SHOULD BE ABOLISHED

EVERYTHING should be ready a quarter of an hour before the lecture is due to start. Punctuality is a sign of respect, and is part of the preparation.

Already two women are waiting, eyeing each other discreetly.

" Is it for gymnastics ? " one of them asks me, obviously ill-informed.

" I shall be talking to you in a moment," I reply, inviting them meanwhile to come into the room where the lecture is to be given. They sit down . . . at the very end of the bench, in the corner farthest from the table. I wait a while, and then ask them if they have to sit right in the corner as a punishment. We laugh about it.

At the appointed time we are still short of two or three patients.

" We shall wait a few minutes if you don't mind. It is not always easy for you ladies to get away; in addition, this is your first attendance, and you don't know that we mean a time when we fix it."

Thus the preliminary steps are taken.

I invite them to make themselves comfortable. They should not feel uneasy, nor feel too hot or too cold; in fact, nothing should hamper them. I explain why this should be so; discomfort means distraction, which would interfere with assimilating the contents of the lecture. This would be unfortunate.

We fix a time and date for the next lecture. I take advantage of this to see their registration book and find out whether they have looked at it.

This book will allow them to record faithfully their attendance at each lecture. There is a page specially set aside for this purpose.

" Faithfully " is the operative word. It is not just a formality, or some form to fill in. This book is claimed back when they are admitted to the labour wards. The record of attendance at lectures is checked and, if for some reason the patient has missed one of them, we know which one straight away and we can take appropriate steps to remedy this.

By then the latecomers have arrived, entering shyly at the back. Once more I invite them to move nearer. The lecture starts.

My lecture today will be fairly long, and I must apologise about this, but it has to be so. I want to tell you why there has been such a thing as pain in childbirth; why and how it can be abolished.

The lecture will therefore be a theoretical one, so that there will not be a class on exercises after this. Exercises will be started after the lecture on breathing. I would like to make it clear that these exercises have nothing whatsoever to do with gymnastics or physical culture. These exercises are straightforward, and in practising them you need no material, nor any special room. They are closely related to the demands made by pregnancy and delivery.

There is another important point as well, which must be clear. This is the " spirit in which you must understand the nature of your preparation ".

These lectures are not meant to be solemn, and you have already realised that. You must look upon them as a method of collaboration between you and us, as team work, in which *everyone* has something to *learn*, to say and to do.

This collaboration does not end with your training—it is carried on into the labour ward. The medical staff looking after you has been selected. It is well versed in the principles and practice of the approach. It will ensure its teaching and its practical application.

It is in your interest to ask questions. You must not be in the dark about anything, and you should always leave here with clear-cut ideas. It would be quite natural for anyone not to understand, straight away and completely, the theoretical principles that will be enunciated. If that is the case do not hesitate to say so; you must not make it a question of pride. There is no such thing as a stupid question; so there will be no unpleasant answers.

Physiology is that branch of science which deals with all the phenomena concerning life, and which seeks to understand them as well as explain them. A part of physiology is devoted to the nervous system; or, if you prefer, to the functions of the nervous system.

We shall now talk about the views that have been held and taught about the physiology of the nervous system for a long time. They were the views of Bichat.

Since Bichat, the orthodox teaching has been that our body had two nervous systems. This is true enough, but it was held that these two systems were independent, quite independent and separate. They were autonomous and unable to exert an influence on one another. All this you have been taught at school.

In fact, you were taught that there was (a) a cerebro-spinal nervous system, and (b) a vegetative or visceral nervous system, and you had to learn what were the functions of these two nervous systems.

The cerebro-spinal system (that is, the brain and spinal cord) is the system responsible for voluntary movement and sensation.

It is by virtue of this system that a human being or an animal can communicate or keep in touch with his surroundings. These surroundings are called his external environment. What allows us to keep in touch with this environment are our sensory organs.

Through them we can pick up and interpret all the excitations, all the stimuli that emanate from our external environment. In fact, these stimuli are perceived by them, relayed along nervous pathways to the brain, where they are analysed, associated and grouped together (or synthetised).

There result, in the brain of man or animal, connected reactions which give rise to a certain activity, a certain behaviour, a certain attitude—a response—corresponding to these stimuli. By means of this response we remain in equilibrium with the requirements of our external environment.

This state of exchange was said to be maintained *essentially* by this cerebro-spinal system. This and only this was its purpose.

Side by side, completely separate from this cerebro-spinal system, there functioned another nervous system: the visceral nervous system.

You were taught at school that this system governed the life of our internal organs and that this was its unique role. Our heart, lungs, liver, stomach, intestines, kidneys, glands, etc., depended on it.

And what about the uterus, you may ask? Well, the uterus too was governed by this system, and your uterus at this very moment shelters your future child.

So which of the two systems is going to influence childbirth?

The visceral nervous system and, according to the above views, only the visceral nervous system. So it was impossible to see how an act, or how a woman's behaviour could have any effect on either the progress or the performance of her labour.

So it could be conceived that pain was part of childbirth, that it was ingrained for ever in woman's make-up, and that she should accept it and suffer it. These views on the physiology of the nervous system are not correct. It is to another man of science, another physiologist, that we must be grateful for proof of the contrary. His name must be familiar to many of you and you were probably told about him at school. He is Pavlov.

Unfortunately, to many schoolgirls the memory of Pavlov is linked with a dog that salivates, and no more. We shall see soon that the name of Pavlov implies a " little more " than a dog that salivates.

From the start of his work (1879—which is not very recent) Pavlov disagreed with Bichat. He felt that no independent functional activity existed in our system. He looked upon the body as a whole, closely integrated and indivisible, in which the equilibrium and development of each organ or system depended on the equilibrium of that whole.

When he talked about unity he meant the unity of the individual's body proper—that is, his own environment, called the internal environment—and the unity of that internal environment with the individual's surroundings, or external environment.

The responsibility of reaching a constant equilibrium was left to the nervous system, which had to maintain the unity between internal and external environment.

Pavlov went further; he argued that the whole nervous system was under the control or the supervision of a superior centre—that is, the brain. He felt that the brain had the property of reacting and answering in a precise manner to *information* received from its own environment as well as from the external environment. The activities of the brain were therefore all-important.

At this stage let me draw your attention to an important fact. I have just spoken about *information* which the brain receives.

Pavlov held that there were two possible methods of information:

1. Direct information, or stimuli perceived by means of our sense organs. This he has called the *first system of signalisation.*

2. Indirect information, again stimuli directly perceived by our sense organs, but recording reality through some other medium—namely, the spoken and the written word.

After numerous observations, Pavlov reached the conclusion that words could take the place of any direct stimulus and replace it. Hence he called language the *second system of signalisation.*

These were the two theories held; that of Bichat, as I said, was wrong, while that of Pavlov was correct.

Does this satisfy you?

No—and you are quite right.

I have so far made firm statements, and you may not believe me. But rest assured, we shall never try to persuade you. Persuasion is a word that finds no place in our teaching. On the contrary, we shall proceed, with the help of demonstration, by offering proof of what we have said or we are going to say. So our teaching will keep its objective character, and right now I shall tell you why Pavlov's theory is correct.

When we come into this world we bring with us what are called *reflexes*, and these are said to be *absolute* or *inborn.*

They are elementary reflexes which allow a human being or animal to react in an elementary manner to the necessities and primitive requirements of life; or, to put it in a different way, to the *stable conditions* of the environment in which we live.

These *responses* guarantee the immediate existence or life of the being or animal and its environmental adaptation.

These responses are exhibited because our nervous

system is organised and built for the purpose of guaranteeing these reactions.

This nervous organisation is the fruit of a slow and continuous evolution of the human species.

Let us consider a few examples of absolute reflexes.

A few hours after the birth of your child you feed it—either breast or bottle.

The child will suck, and the sucking reflex will be most vigorous. You will be overwhelmed with tenderness for your baby.

The reflex the child has just displayed was not taught to it. It is an absolute reflex and forms part of the feeding reflex.

Other examples are spitting out a very sour or very bitter food, and moving away from a flame.

They are defence reflexes.

When you came in here a short while ago you were eager to know what the lecture was all about. This is the reflex of investigation, commonly called curiosity. Why? How? What is it?

Let us go back to the first reflex I mentioned—the feeding reflex.

What is true for us is true as well for animals. Take, for example, the case of a little dog; soon after birth it fights for the mother's dugs. This reflex will last right through its life.

As an adult, the dog no longer feeds on its mother's milk; but should you offer him a piece of meat he will jump for it and will eat it.

If you watch that dog closely you will notice that as it exhibits this feeding reflex it is salivating. Dogs of certain breeds have a plentiful supply of saliva and dribble generously. Salivation, therefore, is an accompaniment of this absolute feeding reflex. This is true of man as well.

Pavlov studied the physiology of the nervous system by

using absolute reflexes as the foundation stones of his work.*

He has carried out his experiments on animals, mostly dogs (which, by the way, were very well looked after), using as a basic rule the absolute feeding reflex.

I shall describe one of Pavlov's earliest experiments to you.

You came here to hear about childbirth in humans, and now we are going to talk about dogs! Don't be offended. You will find the transposition to humans easy.

It is very likely that some of you know this experiment already; I think this is yet another reason for you to listen with greater attention to the explanations I shall give.

These explanations, which are not to be found in class textbooks, will allow you to correlate the experiment with the purpose of these lectures—namely, painless childbirth. They will also fix in your mind the fact that Pavlov was a great man, and his memory will tower above recollections of salivary glands.

Pavlov, in his experiments, decided to precede the showing of food to the dog by a stimulus aimed at one of its sense organs. This stimulus bears no relationship to the food of the dog.

Let us suppose that you switch on an electric light before you give the dog food; or you show it a piece of paper— a green piece; or you arrange for a special smell to be given off in the experimental room; or for a whistle to be blown or a bell rung; or even that the animal be scratched at a definite spot on its skin.

It is difficult to see what relationship exists between any of these stimuli on its own and the food given to the dog. They all seem to be quite unrelated to that food.

* " The Cartesian concept on reflexes is our starting point. That this concept is scientific is obvious, since the phenomenon it describes is strictly defined." From Lecture I—in Pavlov's *Studies of the Cerebral Hemispheres.*

Let us choose one of these stimuli. Has any one of you a choice?

We shall precede feeding by blowing the whistle. This is called a *conditional stimulus*, while the food is the *absolute stimulus*.

The dog eats the meat handed to it. At the same time its salivary glands pour out a certain *amount* of saliva of a certain *quality*.

This experiment is repeated with exactly the same sequence some ten, twenty, thirty times. Each time the dog will react in exactly the same manner. But at the thirty-first time, only the whistle is blown.

We then see that our dog reacts just as before; it displays its feeding reflex, with the amount and quality of saliva being exactly what it was previously.

The absolute feeding reflex has become conditioned to a sonorous stimulus—the whistle.

This experiment is not in fact amazing, but yet it must appear strange to you. And really, you have carried it out hundreds of times, even on yourselves; or you may have seen others carry it out, perhaps on animals.*

Those who keep cats, for example, often do not realise that they need do no more than unhook the scissors to cut the string round the meat for the cat to appear on the scene.

And why? I shall give you an explanation that will apply to cats, dogs or human beings.

The noise made by unhooking the scissors, by *corresponding* in time on many occasions with getting out food for the cat, has assumed the value of a *signal for food*; in the same way that the whistle did before.

Keep this question of *signal* well in mind.

If, in the dog, the experiment is carried on, with the whistle but no meat, we shall soon see that the conditioned reflex disappears. The reflex is said to have become

---

* In human beings I often choose traffic lights as an example: green, amber, red, for pedestrians or drivers.

extinguished; that is, the whistle is no longer a signal. There exists no association between the stimulus (of hearing) and food.

Again, repeating the experiment in its original form, we soon see a quick reappearance of the reflex.

Hence such a reflex takes a long time to initiate, vanishes quickly, and forms anew quickly.

But what does all this amount to? Why has the dog shown such a reaction in response to such a stimulus?

I want you to follow attentively now. This part of the lecture will, in fact, give you the clue between this experiment and childbirth.

It is a knowledge of the " alterations " taking place in the nervous system of the dog that allows one to explain and to understand the reactions and behaviour of the dog.

In other words, it is not the behaviour of the dog that influences its nervous system, but just the reverse.

Why do I lay stress on this point? Because these " alterations " in the dog's nervous system are the direct results of stimuli coming from its external environment.

What has been " altered "? The dog from birth possesses this absolute reflex for feeding since it has some nervous organisation that ensures a response. One could say that circuits or well-established channels were present.

But the second reflex—that of salivating when a whistle is blown—was not present at birth.

It was the very conditions under which the experiment was carried out, which, by acting on the dog's nervous system, have influenced the formation or laying down of new circuits or channels called " temporary associations ".

The first circuit is between the dog's hearing and its brain. Within the latter, nervous cells light up and become active. All the cells becoming alert at the same time constitute a " focus of excitation ".

Almost simultaneously another focus of excitation, relating to food, came into being.

As the experiment is repeated over and over again, and as these foci are lit up, the activity set up encroaches little by little on other nervous cells—a " clearing " is forming.

Hence another channel, another association is being laid down. At the thirty-first repetition the path is completed and results in a functional unit. A sound—the blowing of a whistle—has now acquired the property of a signal for feeding.

The circuit being now complete, the conditioned stimulus takes over from the absolute stimulus, which is now of no use, since the former has replaced it and acts with equal effect on the alimentary mechanism of the dog, especially on its salivary glands.

All this means that the behaviour of the dog is but an answer to the state of its environment at a given time. We call this a response activity.

By now you have gathered that our two nervous systems do not work separately; on the contrary, they are intimately connected and mutually supporting. You have also gathered that the temporary association taking place in the brain confirms the leading role played by the latter. The brain analyses, governs, regroups, synthesises and ensures the exact response.

In the second part of the experiment the reflex died out. This is because an association exists so long as the stimuli exist and bear a relationship to each other in time. Otherwise it soon disappears. Once the circuit is open the conditioned stimulus loses its effect.

In the third part of the experiment the reflex is quickly reformed. This is because impressions of the association still remain.

In everyday language we call this memory.

I mentioned this third part of the experiment to you because there are a few of you who have already had children. You have kept impressions of associations formed as the result of one or more deliveries.

If it is possible to condition an experience—that is, create associations as in the first part of the experiment—it is possible to decondition it; that is, destroy the associations as in the second part of the experiment.

Pavlov has shown us how reflexes behave towards each other; how we can strengthen them or destroy them.

In our last lecture, you will be told—this applies specially to those here who have had children already—what to do to prevent old reflexes from reappearing. You will not be told today; it is important that you should have further information to help you grasp the full implication of your action.

We shall now proceed to see how a human organism behaves and reacts in two well-defined sets of circumstances which may arise.

Let us take the best and most favourable one; that of being in good health and in the waking state. At this very moment you know that your heart must be beating, your lungs oxygenating your blood, and that your stomach, liver and other organs must be functioning. But are you aware of their activities? Can you show me the exact boundaries of your liver simply from your awareness of its activities? No! No, because you cannot feel them. This does not mean that such organs cannot feel. In fact, in all our organs streams of excitations continuously emanate from the nervous endings. These streams move along nervous pathways to reach the brain. Their object is to keep the brain informed. It is therefore a method of intelligence, or of signalisation.

Somehow, when we are in good health and fully awake, these streams, on reaching the brain, meet a barrier that holds them back and stops them from penetrating the brain. This is referred to as inhibition, and they are said to be unable to reach the " threshold of perception " of the brain. Why is this so?

We could compare this, quite validly, to electricity. Let

us say that these streams or currents have a potential force of four volts. Let us say that the potential force of the brain is much higher, say, eight to ten volts—the brain being usually of a higher voltage.

It is this higher power that allows it to keep at bay all the excitations coming from internal organs.

Notice that I said " fully awake ". Why " fully awake " ? Because during sleep the brain is on a reduced output, and therefore at a lower potential. At the same time the intensity of excitations leaving internal organs increases; they are no longer held in check with as much power, so that these two forces tend to match each other.

This phenomenon explains why the first indication that labour is starting is most often felt at night.

So much for this; what about the second circumstance?

You know full well that we can discern appreciably and even painfully the working of our internal organs, quite apart from any disease or lesion. A very strong emotional upset is a case in point. For example, a telegram bringing news of the sudden death of a beloved acquaintance would make us go pale, feel sick and giddy, dry our mouth or feel a sensation of painful constriction in our throat or stomach; we feel our heart beat fast, and louder and louder.

These organs suddenly feel pain, but they are not " diseased ". This painful perception can be explained. The stimuli leaving these various organs at the time the telegram was read had their usual intensity (plus four), but they travelled to a brain in a state of diminished activity as the result of a sudden and marked alteration.

This is a well-known phenomenon. The negative character of this emotional shock had influenced the potential force of the brain, lowering it sufficiently to alter the balance of power. The stimuli at a level of four were now strong enough to overcome the threshold of sensitivity of the brain, now, say, at a level of three.

We are dealing here with a sudden and brutal change. But this lack of balance of power can creep in slowly as the result of what is termed microtraumata—that is, many small upsets or shocks. They must be numerous to be effective; acting singly, they make no impression.

If today some small point is bothering you and if by tomorrow everything has settled down, will this small point have upset the equilibrium of your nervous system? No. But if every day, for a year, it bothered you, the summation of these annoyances would exert on your nervous system the same effect as a drop of water falling regularly at the same spot on a hard stone. A few drops—no effect. Millions of drops—a hole. Your disorganised nervous system can no longer guarantee exact responses.

This example of microtraumata bears a close resemblance to the effect made on you by (a) what you may hear; (b) what you may read before or during pregnancy, and directly concerning your pregnancy or delivery.

A slow disorganisation of your nervous system, a slow disturbance of its equilibrium, once started, will soon become more prominent, and will predispose you to the effect of the final shock—here, the first manifestations of labour. We can compare the first contractions to the emotional upset following the receipt of the telegram.

There follows a complete disruption of the equilibrium of the nervous system. These first contractions, though normal in intensity, are nevertheless strong enough to spill over the threshold of perception. From then onwards *contraction becomes a signal for pain.*

Do you talk of "contractions" when you refer to the beginning of labour? Certainly not; you talk of "pains". You would say, in a solemn way, "When I had my first pains".

Your behaviour would then be the reflection of a nervous organisation conforming to some preconceived attitude to pregnancy and labour. It would amount to a collection of harmful conditioned reflexes.

If all this applies to you, it applies just as much to the medical world. It was unusual for us, in talking to you, to speak of contractions. When we used this term, we saw behind it the shadow of pain. Pain was looked upon as essential and necessary. It was a normal physiological manifestation and was classified into two sections, the beneficial and the prejudicial.

Pain was one of the *conditions of labour. So our attitude towards labour was nothing else but the mirror of these views.*

Recapitulating, it was thought that:

1. Pain was a condition of delivery.
2. The two nervous systems were independent of each other.
3. Our cerebro-spinal system was exclusively linked with our surroundings.
4. It could not influence the processes involved in labour.

Hence labour could be seen only in a light that gave the woman a *passive* role. Was it not true that, once a woman was in the delivery room, she had to wait until " it happened "? This was true for you, for midwives, or for women doctors.

After everything I have said today you will appreciate what a colossal mistake this was.

To all of you joining in this preparation delivery will be an *active event*. When you are admitted to our labour ward, you will come in to complete an action. After you have taken full cognizance of your maturity, you will have a chance of *analysing* it, of *controlling* its progress and of *checking up* at each stage the benefit arising from what you have been taught. You will give *impetus* to your delivery by remaining its *driving force*.

How will you achieve this?

I have explained to you how your nervous system has

been slowly but surely disorganised by repeated traumatic episodes. This traumatism hit you very hard; the reason for this lies in your ignorance regarding pregnancy and labour.

This is not meant as a reproach. You were not fortunate enough in your education. When you were at school you were told much about the reproduction of flowers, animals and plants. But absolutely nothing about yourself. When you left school what did you know about yourself? Nothing! What a mistake! A mistake made by the educationalists who have a say in the preparation of schedules of studies, and who have failed you by refusing to teach you and educate you in a rational manner about this topic.

A mistake also for having ignored Pavlov, because they have been blind to the inborn reflex of investigation. This " curiosity " fills every young girl at puberty; it is the same curiosity that arouses her interest in ladies with big stomachs and drives her to talk in confidence to her young friends. She is already trying to find out what is going on. Soon she knows all about it; the good lady has had a baby, she screamed, she was in pain, she lost blood, and she had to keep to her bed.

Childbirth is soon associated with pain and danger. A start has been made; from then onwards childbirth remains linked with pain and danger.

We shall endeavour to make good this blank as quickly as possible. We shall do what should have been done: we shall educate you; because the prophylactic elimination of pain in childbirth is achieved by education.

Your behaviour will then reflect this education, formulated at a higher level of consciousness. It will amount to a new system of nervous organisation, in which new conditioned reflexes are acquired and linked with the requirements of childbirth.

So your reactions will be in keeping with the demands of each phase of delivery and your behaviour will see that you adapt yourself rationally to the phenomenon.

We have begun this education. In the days to come we shall talk to you about the position of your genital organs, as well as the work of those specially involved in delivery. We shall study their relationships and we shall tell you how they function.

You will realise that:

1. These organs are made to hold and shelter the child.
2. After holding and sheltering it, they can expel it.
3. Your pregnancy and delivery are part of your life, being two natural and physiological phenomena.
4. Pain is no more essential to labour than it is to pregnancy, and that it is harmful to delivery as it would be to pregnancy.

We shall then describe in detail what happens during delivery; the organic functional changes and stages that accompany it; the value of these changes; and finally what you should do during each stage and the reason for this response activity—I repeat, *response activity*.

At no time during labour should your actions distract you; on the contrary, they should make you act in full consciousness of your identification with your delivery (through your active participation).

You will no longer approach your delivery as resigned women facing inescapable pain. You will have been handed a stock of information, amply sufficient to allow you to give birth with *full knowledge* and with joy.

Before leaving you today I want to warn you against yourselves. Take good note of this: childbirth without pain does not mean childbirth without effort. Childbirth demands of a woman a great expenditure of energy. You will be asked to put forth great efforts, and you will succeed—provided you have prepared for it.

In that way you will get through; otherwise you will fail.

On top of the lectures you will attend, you will have

some work to do; you will have to revise the theory, assimilate it and put it into practice.

Some women say that childbirth without pain is a question of controlling oneself. Others that where there is a will there is a way. All this is quite incorrect.

To be able to do something, one must learn how to do it. One must know and one must practise. *If we are not acquainted with the laws of nature we cannot use them to our advantage.*

The character of your pregnancy will now change. It is no longer a passive endless wait as of old; it has become active. It is a study of analysis and control, as, for example, of the movements of the child, of the contractions of the uterus, and of various exercises.

You will move from pregnancy to childbirth as from one state to the next; and this transition is made the easier for being the better informed. And do not forget that your best attainments are acquired in the school of practice.

ANATOMICAL AND PHYSIOLOGICAL RELATIONSHIPS BETWEEN BREATHING, PREGNANCY AND DELIVERY

PLAN OF THE COURSE

RECAPITULATION of the teachings at school on respiratory function.

Role of oxygen in life.

Stressing the constant relationship between cardiac rhythm and respiratory rhythm.

Mechanism of breathlessness.

JUSTIFICATION OF BREATHING EXERCISES

1. They allow the conscious appraisal of the *physical existence* of anatomical relations between the organs directly or indirectly concerned with labour.

These relations are further elaborated in the second part of the course.

2. They amount to a physical training for an event that has a definite physical aspect.

It is a training with a view to coping with all eventualities by (*a*) building good muscular tone, and (*b*) controlling its effects.

3. The gaseous exchanges, richer in oxygen, improve the pulmonary ventilation of the future mother. The new oxygen demands created by pregnancy are met with, as are those of labour.

(A) DURING PREGNANCY

A better pulmonary ventilation helps to ensure adequate oxygenation in the child. The great changes taking place in the transformation of fats and calcium into living matter suggest that more numerous and more intense expenditures of energy result, calling for greater oxygenation.

The woman gains in weight and accumulates fats more easily, so her muscles have more work to do. She consumes more, so that once more the answer is oxygen.

(B) DURING LABOUR

A great expenditure of energy is accompanied by intense combustion, requiring a constant supply of oxygen to the main organs or systems in action, such as:

1. The nervous system, above all the brain, which analyses, controls and directs.
2. The uterus, during its numerous internal contractions.
3. Muscular efforts at all stages of labour and chiefly during delivery, when the *pressure of the abdominal muscles is added to that of uterine contraction.*

The exertion made by the woman is considerable, though lasting only for relatively short periods. But *should it be inadequate*, or should the parturient show no adaptation and, above all, should her *respiratory response* fail to appear quickly enough to offer compensation, then there follows a quickening of the pulse, breathlessness, tiredness and perhaps even collapse.

This is an almost classical picture of labour as it used to be.

What were the consequences resulting from this state of affairs?

(*a*) For the mother, not grave, only that she will be longer going back to her usual activities.

(*b*) For the child the consequences can be more serious when we consider the unfavourable conditions that are thrust upon it during labour. Labour creates a delicate situation in the life of a child.

During dilatation the uterus contracts vigorously on it. During delivery it is forcefully expulsed from the uterus. It has to navigate a canal, fairly narrow and flanked by bony walls. It is said—it is a fact—that delivery is traumatic for it.

Such little traumata should not be allowed to become too numerous; hence the necessity to find proper means of shortening labour. Whether the dilatation stage of labour or the delivery be considered, it still remains that the child must receive a constant and sufficient supply of oxygen. This means a good or a bad start in life for the child; and such a responsibility falls mostly on the mother.

Were women capable of facing labour actively in 1951? Are they all being offered this advantage now?

This latter question is answered by preparing the mother for childbirth by the psychoprophylactic method.

Such responsibilities are accepted and shared.

The patient undertakes her labour when well-informed and knows why some processes help its progress. Furthermore, responsibilities are shared through the *help* she knows she will receive.

The medical staff, versed in the principles of the method and trained to apply it, must:

(a) *Watch* the progress of labour from an obstetric angle.

(b) Keep the woman informed of such progress as well as *be kept informed* by her.

(c) Reinforce the education of the woman; that is, everything she has learnt during her preparation— her acquired capital of useful reflexes.

In addition the woman should be in a comfortable room of her own, and we must make certain that she artificially oxygenates her blood from a certain stage in her labour.

THE MECHANISM OF BREATHING

The diaphragm is described in its role as an essential muscle of respiration. Its situation, attachments and

Action of the diaphragm during the stage of delivery

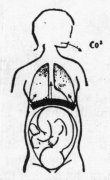 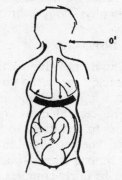

1. At rest and during expiration, the diaphragm does not press on the uterus

2. Holding the breath after inspiration causes the diaphragm to press on the uterus, thus adding this pressure to that of uterine contraction

The three forces that act on the child and add up to delivery

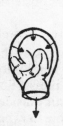 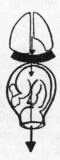 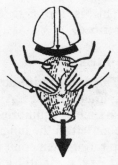

1. Uterine contraction

2. Uterine contraction *and* action of the diaphragm

3. Uterine contraction *and* action of the diaphragm *and* belt-like action of abdominal muscles

Figure 8

relations are mentioned: chiefly its indirect relationship to the fundus of the uterus.

Its physiology is discussed.

(A) INSPIRATION

This is not due to the direct action of the lungs. The thoracic cage is the go-between. It is this cage which, by increasing its volume, pulls the lungs out with it.

The central dome of the diaphragm flattens out and comes to rest itself, to press down, on the abdominal contents. The peripheral muscular fibres—those that surround this central dome—come into action next. They impart to the ribs fairly complex movements which, by adding their effect to those of the diaphragmatic dome, lead to an increase in width of the three diameters of the thoracic cage.

These diameters are: (1) the vertical one; (2) the one from front to back; (3) the one from side to side, or transverse one.

It must be stressed that in the pregnant woman *the diaphragm comes to rest on the fundus of the uterus*.

This is the *first important function* which must be described.

(B) EXPIRATION

This is a passive act. The thoracic cage collapses as the diaphragm relaxes. Air escapes freely from the lungs until such time as equilibrium is reached between the pressure of the air left in the lungs and the pressure of the air outside. Expiration then comes to a stop, but it is possible to expel part of the air still left in the lungs. This part is what is called complementary air.

(C) FORCEFUL EXPIRATION

This is achieved by bringing the abdominal muscles into action.

Let us point out that these are the very muscles that the woman uses during delivery.

A study of the geography of these muscles makes for a better understanding of the movements they can induce, during contraction, in the bones into which they are inserted. This is the *second important function* to be described.

The superior insertions of the abdominal muscles are in the inferior part of the thoracic cage. Their inferior insertions are in the upper edges of the pelvis.

When the pelvis is fixed, these muscles exert a vertical pull on the thoracic cage; they act then as expiratory muscles.

When the ribs have reached their lowermost position, should these abdominal muscles contract further they will elevate the pelvis, causing it to tilt backwards and upwards.

This elevating of the pelvis is accompanied by a favourable straightening of the curves in the vertebral column.

ADVANTAGES OF BREATHING LESSONS

(a) On the diaphragm. Its tone increases and the chest expansion improves. A better discipline of its action is obtained.

(b) On the abdominal muscles. Their tone increases, and with it a greater precision in their action.

So we can end by saying that with stronger abdominal muscles the woman will furnish more efficient and powerful efforts during delivery, also such efforts will be correctly applied. Hence the time spent on delivery will be considerably decreased.

PREPARATORY EXERCISES

They will act as a link between the theoretical teachings and physical reality.

They will allow the woman to analyse and study the anatomical relations described from her own personal point of view.

They consist of:

1. A deep inspiration, through the nose if possible.
2. Expiration in two stages:
   (a) Passive stage. With mouth open, to let air escape freely from the lungs until equilibrium is reached.
   (b) Active stage. Use abdominal muscles. Imagine a burning candle some 2 feet away. Blow on it to bend the flame *without putting it out.*

Why? Because the resistance caused by the pinching of the lips can only be overcome by a certain force. The flame is bent over a certain period of time and the lungs are emptied of complementary air. Hence the need to contract the abdominal muscles with some force over some length of time.

Position—on one's back, on a couch.

Number of times—three times a day for some three to five minutes.

Alter the respiratory exchanges (inspiration and expiration accordingly) from five to nine times per minute.

Do not overdo either inspiration or expiration.

Carefully *analyse* the relations described.

Inspiration → diaphragm → uterine fundus → vertical compression.

Expiration → abdominal muscles → collapse of ribs → lateral compression of uterus and elevation of the pelvis.

LECTURE III

FOETAL MOVEMENTS. UTERINE CONTRACTIONS DURING PREGNANCY. NEUROMUSCULAR EDUCATION

FOETAL MOVEMENTS

DURING pregnancy you have two natural means of ascertaining the anatomy and position of the uterus inside your abdomen.

You have already come across these two means. They are the movements of the foetus and the contractions of the uterus.

I suppose that you have all felt the child move. You must have certainly remarked on these movements.

In the first instance, they happen at any time, and in any position without any warning. They have a lawless temperament.

Secondly, they are shortlived—four to five seconds.

Thirdly, they are localised; that is, they take place in one spot in the abdomen at a time.

This spot is not always the same. In fact movements take place anywhere inside the uterus.

Fourthly, they are at times very strong.

How can we exploit these foetal movements and analyse their relationship to the uterus, if they are shortlived and lawless?

This does not seem to be an easy task. But, fortunately, since our last lecture you have certainly noticed something interesting.

While carrying out your breathing exercises, or shortly after, have you not felt your baby move more vigorously and for longer? That is so!

Well, everything is simpler now. Since you know that

your baby is going to move, then, you can become more attentive. You will seek to understand these movements and to study them carefully, chiefly in respect of their relationship to the uterus.

Since they do not appear always at the same place you should, studying them at each occasion, slowly delineate the contours of the uterus. It will assume a shape, it will cease to be some vague mass inside your abdomen. You will soon know it well.

Your uterus keeps contracting during pregnancy. Physically speaking, a contraction is felt as a hardening of the abdomen. Women say clearly that they have the impression that for a while their abdomen feels harder. During that contraction its shape alters.

Let us now study these contractions, so as to derive some benefit from them.

They have features that differentiate them from foetal movements and will allow you to recognise the contractions of labour.

However, they have something in common with foetal movements. They, too, are lawless and are felt at any time; but, contrary to foetal movements, they are not localised. It is the uterus as a whole that becomes " hard ". Finally, a contraction lasts twenty to sixty seconds.

These differences are, in principle, sufficiently marked for you to differentiate the two. But, since some of you may not have picked out these contractions, I shall give you a further clue.

Palpate your abdomen and rest your hand on it for some time. Sooner or later you will feel it become harder. It will stay hard for twenty to sixty seconds, this being the time a contraction lasts, since you are then feeling a contraction.

But you do not know yet how to derive benefit from these contractions; that is, how to study them, analyse them in yourselves, and grasp their reality.

As they are inconstant, your research work may be

complicated. However, you have certainly discovered that they are felt when you change position, as when you lie down to sleep. Choose this moment, by far the most favourable one. Try to find where in your abdomen contractions start; how they increase in strength and reach their climax; how long they last and how they subside before disappearing.

If you devote time to such analysis you will reach labour knowing exactly what a contraction is, and you will not be surprised by the start of labour. Once you know their span, the way they start, they develop and they disappear, you will respond to these contractions without difficulty.

You will have benefited by experience which is rich in practical knowledge.

These contractions differ from those of labour in that the latter are regular and are of greater intensity.

PLAN OF THE NEUROMUSCULAR EDUCATION

What is meant by muscular proprioception, and what is the nervous mechanism of this proprioception?

A motor order leaves the brain and is transmitted to a muscle which obeys it by contracting. The stimulation of the nervous end-organs which this muscle contains is passed back to the brain, where it falls upon its sensory perception. Muscular contraction is the work of the brain conveying itself as a positive effect from a motor point of view. It is this nervous process which makes it possible for an individual to pick exactly the site occupied by one of his muscles, and to be conscious of its effect, both in strength and in direction.

When the motor order is withdrawn—that is, when the motor centres become extinguished—the muscle stops working immediately.

The muscle is resting; there is muscular relaxation. This relaxation is the work of the brain conveying itself as a negative effect from a motor point of view.

Muscular relaxation is thus an active phenomenon and not a passive one as far as the brain is concerned.

THE ROLE OF NEUROMUSCULAR EDUCATION IN PAINLESS CHILDBIRTH

This is but *one* of the items of the preparation. Its aim is to give the woman a theoretical and practical knowledge of the following:

1. The muscles that play a useful part in the rational fulfilment of her childbirth; rehearsing their labour, so that care and economy in fulfilment result.

2. The muscles that play no useful part and which are likely to have an antagonistic effect on contraction or be prejudicial to the work of the uterus.

The woman learns how to *hold* these muscles in a state of relaxation; and she endeavours to obtain the best possible *motor co-ordination.* She rehearses useful movements, favourable positions and postures that are an advantage at certain times.

This knowledge, made up of new reflexes acquired and put into practice during the uterine contractions of labour, prevents any disorganisation in the patient, expressed as restlessness and motor inco-ordination.

We try to impart to the woman *during her pregnancy* some form of discipline. This discipline amounts to the formation of centres of excitation and of new connections at brain level.

At the very moment when the first contraction appears the woman gets the maximum functional efficiency out of her brain, and raises the threshold of painful perception by practising all the reflexes she acquired during her preparation.

Let it be recalled that this efficiency stays linked with a knowledge of the reasons behind it.

Again, the words " *at the very moment* " should be stressed, because it is most important that the response reaction should coincide with the first sign of a contraction.

EXERCISES

Position. Lying down, usually on the back; at other times on the sides and eventually sitting up.

1. Start with respiratory exercises. Breathe in, breathe out, blow on the candle (passive interval serves no purpose). Do it two, three or four times.

2. Tone up the muscles (and become conscious of them) by contracting them in turn, small groups at a time, strenuously but not with exaggeration.

3. Stop all contraction and stay relaxed.

4. Control over this muscular relaxation is maintained.

5. End the exercises with the same respiratory ones as at the start.

Progress. Check it during the first four or five days by the successive mobilisation of different parts of the body.

Do not interfere with this mobilisation by either helping it or opposing it.

Next, first elaboration. During the check mobilise one segment of a limb, not always the same. Do this each day for four or five days.

Then, last elaboration. During the check mobilise two segments of a limb simultaneously and keep varying the segments.

By studying this progress carefully, it is possible for the woman first to differentiate, and next to dissociate, anything that has a positive effect from anything that has a negative one as far as the motor system is concerned. So much so that by the time labour is reached the woman can induce a muscle to work on *its own*, while the others which do not need to work are *maintained* in a state of relaxation.

During delivery, for example, her apprenticeship will have taught her how to contract her abdominal muscles while she keeps the muscles of her pelvic floor relaxed. There will be no obstruction to overcome forcibly; hence the duration of delivery will be shortened accordingly.

Sequence. Four times a day; a maximum of five minutes each time.

LABOUR

A<small>T</small> the term of pregnancy, which, let it be recalled, is always only an *approximate* date, varying as much as ten to fifteen days either way, labour will start.

Several manifestations may have preceded it, such as:

(*a*) Irregular contractions, erratic both in intensity and in duration.

(*b*) Heaviness of the lower abdomen.

(*c*) Lumbar ache.

(*d*) Frequent desire to pass water.

(*e*) Some degree of insomnia and loss of appetite.

(*f*) Hyper- or hypoactivity and, finally, symptoms which will remind many women of the onset of menstruation.

Then, under the impulse of some major upheaval in the body, brought about by her mental, biological and nervous factors, labour will start around the 270th day of pregnancy, and will present itself in three main ways:

1. Loss of the mucous plug with loss of blood-stained fluid.

2. Loss of a variable amount of clear, viscous fluid, following the breaking of the pocket of water.

3. Chiefly, the presence of regular rhythmic contractions.

The hallmark of labour is uterine contraction, and its purpose is to dilate the neck of the uterus steadily to allow the delivery of the child.

How Does Labour Work?

In three main stages:

1. " Taking up " of the neck of the uterus.
2. Dilatation of that neck.
3. Delivery: (*a*) osseous component; (*b*) muscular component; (*c*) presentation of the child at the external vaginal orifice.

All these stages take place in a precise order and by the action of a sole mechanism: *uterine contraction.*

What Is Uterine Contraction?

It is a muscular contraction of a similar nature to the contraction of the biceps when the forearm is brought against the upper arm, or to the contraction of the calf muscles during walking or running. But the biceps or calf muscles come under the influence of will and their contraction is voluntary; in the case of the uterus the contraction is involuntary. This contraction, according to the case, can take place under favourable or unfavourable conditions. What we seek to obtain during painless childbirth are the best local and general conditions possible. Such conditions can only prevail if the cortex of the woman is in a state of equilibrium; this would be the case in the woman who knows how to harmonise her uterine contraction with the various functions of her body.

Uterine contraction is felt as a slow and progressive hardening of the uterine muscle, accompanied by a modification of the whole abdominal contents. This process can be externally appreciated by a hand resting on the abdomen. Uterine contraction could be compared to the ebb and flow of a tide. The phase of contraction would be the succession of waves in the rising tide; the intermediate even stage of maximum contraction would be the stagnation of water at high tide; then the stage of waning of the

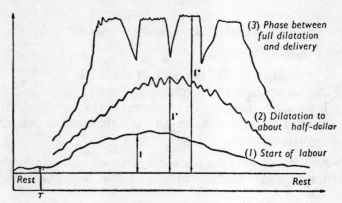

Figure 9

*Kymograph of the changes in the nature of the contraction
at various stages of labour*

*T, T': muscular tone
I, I', I": intensity of the contraction*

contraction would be the ebbing tide. Depicting this picture on a time scale we have:

Waxing of contraction: rising tide.
Apogee of contraction: slack water.
Waning of contraction: ebbing tide.

Between each contraction there is a period of rest that allows the uterus and the body to recuperate and re-establish its equilibrium.

FEATURES OF CONTRACTION

In normal labour (and we always talk about normal labour) the contractions get more frequent and more intense, and this is essential in allowing the woman to *adapt* herself. The human body can pass from a state of rest to one of activity only by going through consecutive stages. Any sudden and quick activity is ill received by the body; on the other hand, gradual adaptation is the ideal state of affairs. This is one of the reasons why, in certain cases (e.g. deeply engaged head), the woman finds difficulty in adapting herself to this new state. If, however, the contractions are at first twenty minutes apart, then fifteen, then ten, etc., adaptation is an easy process in a well-prepared woman.

In normal labour, once " uterine contraction " has become established, it will recur regularly until delivery of the child. Depending on the case, it can be of varying intensity and varying duration.

The diagram (Figure 9) shows the kymographic recording of uterine contractions at various stages:

1. At the start of labour.
2. When dilatation has reached the size of a half-dollar.
3. Stage preceding delivery.

The effects of uterine contractions are:
1. To draw up the cervix.
2. To cause the cervix to dilate.
3. To expel the child.

THE CONDITIONS ESSENTIAL TO THE NORMAL PHYSIOLOGY OF UTERINE CONTRACTION

1. Good oxygenation. This can be obtained in two ways:

(*a*) A diminution in oxygen consumption, which is achieved by the whole body being at rest through *controlled neuromuscular relaxation*. Only the uterus is at work during the taking up and dilatation of the cervix. By keeping the other muscles at rest, the patient economises on oxygen and at the same time reduces the production of waste products. The total effect is a diminution in her respiratory efforts.

(*b*) A constant and regular supply of oxygen through a respiratory rhythm in harmony with uterine contraction.

2. Satisfactory elimination of waste products responsible for such important symptoms as tiredness, cramp, increased muscular tone and tetany, all of which induce pain.

If a muscle at work receives a supply of oxygen according to its need and eliminates all its waste products in a regular manner, then the optimum conditions for it to carry on its effort for long periods at a time will prevail locally.

3. *A good cortical control* is the most important factor required. It will ensure that the two conditions mentioned above are obtained, and it will co-ordinate the work of the uterus with the various processes in the body of which it is unquestionably part and parcel.

The brain can be compared to the head engineer in a perfect central power station.

At first the contractions are weak and the woman may hardly be aware of them, more so if she has had (as is often the case) irregular contractions during the last weeks of pregnancy. There must be a certain number of regular contractions within a definite time before a woman should think in terms of the start of labour. She will have decidedly rejected the association of contraction and pain to enjoy the contrary feeling that these contractions are but the start of a labour which will help her bring into this world, under the best possible conditions, the child she is carrying.

Regularity of rhythm is one of the hall-marks of the contractions of labour, and disappears only in abnormal cases. Subsequently the contractions become progressively more frequent and stronger and allow the woman to adapt herself slowly to her new state.

What are the effects of the uterine contractions? They act on the longitudinal muscle fibres of the uterus while the cervix is taken up and dilates.

First, while the cervix is being taken up, it will work by pulling up the external opening of that cervix, thereby slowly shortening it (total length of about 2 inches) and causing this external opening to merge with the internal one so as to leave only a ring. Hence the cervix will in turn become 2, $1\frac{1}{2}$, 1 and $\frac{1}{2}$ inches long and eventually disappear.

This marks the beginning of the second phase of labour, or phase of true dilatation.

Next, during dilatation these uterine contractions will act on this ring in such a way that it slowly opens like a diaphragm, being at first the diameter of a dime, and then that of a quarter, half-dollar, silver dollar, the size of a half-fist, eventually that of a fist, by which time full dilatation has been reached. At this very moment the back of the head (occiput) of the child will be capped by the cervix, as by a crown. The head, meeting no further obstacle, will descend within the bony pelvis and this will constitute the stage of delivery.

Each uterine contraction, in its effect on the cervix, is helped by a mechanism strictly depending on itself. In fact, during each contraction, the uterine cavity shrinks and presses upon the child. The latter in turn will move in the direction of least resistance, which happens to be through the cervix; and its occiput, being the most perfect of ovoids, exerts on the cervix a steady pressure that brings about the shortening and dilatation of the latter. So we are back to one and the same phenomenon, namely, that uterine contraction has two effects which add up to produce the same result.

These two stages of labour can last, on the average, eight to twelve hours in a primigravida, or three to six hours in a multipara. This means a *big effort* on the part of the parturient, since, though barely active physically, she must remain active on the *cortical side* so as to control, co-ordinate and subsequently direct the progress of her labour. She must be aware of this effort and do her utmost to spare her energy. Breathing and neuromuscular relaxation will be used only deliberately and separately. This means that it is not a question of teaching the woman, during her training, that she must breathe rapidly and shallowly or relax systematically during such and such a stage of labour; far from it—she must remain the sole judge of when and how to do it, keeping constantly in mind the importance of avoiding any unnecessary fatigue. These lengthy stages will, therefore, entail a demand for constant control with a minimum of physical activity, chiefly at such times as the contractions become crowded together and strong.

The end of the stage of dilatation is characterised by a discomfort felt by most women, save those who, it seems, fall in the category of the well-balanced types. This discomfort is a physiological phenomenon; it corresponds to a tug-of-war between the head seeking to enter the pelvis (pre-delivery) and the yet incompletely dilated cervix. The uterine contraction loses its regular rhythm of the stage of dilatation; it is no longer the type of contraction that causes dilatation, and is not yet the type that leads to expulsion of the child.

It is at this moment, above all, that the second system of signalisation becomes indispensable. The choice of words used will have all its effect, and the woman will succeed in rapidly reaching the stage of delivery proper.

These two stages should be as easy as they are short, this being the attribute of a good presentation and a supple cervix. Any other state constitutes a situation which the woman will overcome more or less easily, according to her nervous equilibrium.

DELIVERY

The stage of delivery is that final stage of labour which causes the child to leave the uterine cavity and pass through the pelvis of the mother. Two phases can be distinguished:

1. The osseous phase.
2. The muscular phase, divided into (a) the perineal phase; (b) the delivery proper.

This stage of labour will depend on the action of two factors—uterine contraction and the added efforts of the mother.

The uterine contraction of this stage differs from those of the preceding stages by the nature of their identity. It is the most powerful of all uterine contractions because all strata of fibres of the uterine muscle are brought into play. This being the case, the contractions direct their action along a resultant line lying in the axis of the pelvis and seek to empty the uterus of its contents and push them through the pelvic cavity with varying degrees of friction.

If these contractions act on their own they may prove to be inadequate and so protract the stage of delivery. This is why the mother's efforts at delivering herself must be co-ordinated with uterine contractions.

The mother's efforts will consist in a deep inspiration which will steady the diaphragm against the fundus of the uterus, thereby affording it support, followed by a contraction of the thoracic and upper abdominal muscles to form an abdominal belt around the uterus. These pressure effects are thus added to the force of contraction of the uterus. Pushed by the coupling of these combined effects— the one involuntary (uterine contraction), the other voluntary (mother's muscular efforts)—the child will make headway through the pelvic cavity.

The child's head will be well flexed at first during the osseous phase—a phase demanding great physical effort on the part of the mother. Then the head extends during the muscular perineal phase, at which time the woman is asked to display enormous efforts of control with diminished physical effort. The head, therefore, pivots around the pubic symphysis, which acts as a hinge.

This stage takes place under the command of the obstetrician-in-charge. One parturient has defined this very well: " The obstetrician was the conductor; I was the first violin."

Here, more than at any other time, words play an important role, somewhat similar to those of the athletic coach. *They should be precise, convincing and stimulating in order to be effective.* One should choose words that have been used during the preparation. The inflexion of the voice should vary according to the woman. It should be kind or firm, incisive or soft, quiet, and never hurried. The obstetrician should always remember the old saying: " The obstetrician must know how to bestow his time, and do so graciously."

How is this stage to be managed? The woman, having settled down to her delivery, will inform the obstetrician each time she has a contraction. He will then direct her thus: " Breathe in, blow out "; then " Breathe in, hold it, pull on the bars, bring your chest out and push well down."

If necessary, during the same contraction, the obstetrician may direct the woman to empty her lungs by getting her to breathe out and then breathe in fully, and then hold it before pushing down.

Once the contraction is over, the obstetrician directs her to relax completely and regain her strength for the next contraction. During this period, demanding much effort, the woman, if she so wishes, can have a drink between contractions or have her face wiped with a moist sponge and, if she needs it, she can be given oxygen.

When the head, having dilated the perineum, presents itself at the outlet of the vagina and slowly dilates it, the woman should push more steadily, keeping time with the obstetrician encouraging her in a crescendo fashion.

When finally, under the pressure exerted by the occiput and with the perfect control of her perineal muscles, the external vaginal orifice is sufficiently dilated, the woman will adopt a *panting type of breathing* while the midwife deals with the delivery of the head.

As the midwife slips the mother's perineum down the child's face she will say successively at regular intervals: " The roots of the hair, the forehead, the eyes, the nose, the mouth, the chin." Then, giving the mother a breathing space of five to ten seconds, she will ask her to push down so as to bring the nearer shoulder of the child under her pubic symphysis. She then brings out that arm and rests it on the mother, affording her the first emotional contact she has with her child. She then brings out the other arm and pulls the child into view; and very often, as the mother rights herself, she will hold out her arms to pick up her child, her face lighting up with extreme delight and deep pride.

The birth proper is now over, and in a further seven to ten minutes the placenta separates and is in turn delivered.

This stage, markedly shortened in the prepared woman as compared to the unprepared one, can be summarised thus:

Osseous phase: great physical effort.
Perineal phase: great physical effort, plus control.
Delivery phase: control only.

These three phases are the result of a perfect training and a complete harmony between all those taking part in this creative achievement. Here rest the true laurels of the second system of signalisation in its most valuable application.

This stage may be easier in the primigravida than in the multipara, who may have been deeply branded (a tenacious conditioned reflex, resulting from a powerful stimulus, even if it happened once) by the sudden arrival of the head on the perineum, bringing back recollections of her previous deliveries.

In this group of women a half-success in her first experience of " painless childbirth " will pave the way for more favourable circumstances, making her next labour a complete success.

In concluding, we will say that painless childbirth cannot be, for the time being, a way out for the laziness or complacency either of women or of those helping them during labour. *It must be a co-ordinated effort based on harmony and enthusiasm.*

BEHAVIOUR OF THE WOMAN DURING THE FIRST STAGE

GIVE the classical description of the physiological changes leading to the slow and progressive elimination of anything standing in the way of exit of the child; namely, the mucous plug, the membranes and the non-dilated cervix.

Give an idea of the total time needed; a relative value for the woman.

Give an idea of the duration of real labour; that is, the sum of the length of the contractions.

THE CONTRACTIONS

Note:

Duration.

Intervals between them—at the beginning and at the end.

Intensity of a contraction; an ascending curve in the first half of its duration, a descending one in the second half.

Intensity of contractions; stronger at the end than at the beginning.

Words used to denote the diameter of the dilating cervix: dime, quarter, half-dollar, silver dollar, half-fist, fist.

Physical signs associated with contractions, such as: hardening of the abdomen; change in shape of the uterus, which becomes shorter; feeling of something pulling at the level of the pubis; heaviness above the pubis; pressure of the head on the internal os (orifice) of the cervix.

These first two stages can only be studied provided the organic changes corresponding to them are appreciated.

Stress the necessity of spotting and analysing contractions during pregnancy; here prophylaxis means knowledge. And, since childbirth is but a change in the nature of the pregnancy, the latter must be fully grasped to arrive at an understanding of the former. Hence the conditions governing pregnancy will be the same governing childbirth. We cannot say this too often.

GENERAL BEHAVIOUR : SOME SET PROBLEMS

1. BETWEEN CONTRACTIONS

(A) WITHOUT PREPARATION

How did women behave during labour? What did they do?—Nothing.

What was on their mind?—The next contraction.

Hence the dread of the next contraction, which meant a deepening of the rent in the energy relationship and a lowering of the threshold of perception of the brain.

A contraction was the signal of pain; and pain there resulted.

(B) WITH PREPARATION

Contraction is accompanied by the normal perception of a sensation; it is no longer the signal for pain; there no longer exists a physiological conflict. The proof comes from the woman because she has responded to it and she has adapted herself, while the energy relationship and the nervous equilibrium are kept up solely by full and active consciousness.

So, between contractions, the main concern of the woman will be to show a better response to the demands of labour. Her next concern will be to make good use of the intervals between contractions, by avoiding unnecessary efforts and recuperating herself to a maximum in the minimum time available.

2. During Contractions

Recapitulate Lecture III.

To ensure that pain is not felt, the excitations leaving the uterus, *regardless of their intensity*, must not cross the threshold of sensitive perception of the brain.

For this to be the case the woman must reach labour in a perfect state of nervous equilibrium, then maintain this state by putting into practice her acquired knowledge, helped by the medical attendant or attendants.

Response activity depends on needs and on the functional state of active organs—chiefly the uterus. It must be given the best possible conditions for its work; not only should it not be hindered, but its contractions should be helped along.

During a contraction the following are observed:

(*a*) *Shallow* breathing, which restrains the movements of the diaphragm, limits its downstroke and prevents or diminishes the vertical compression of the uterine fundus and its appendages, which are all very sensitive to heavy pressure. (The woman has already found out during pregnancy that deep inspiration can be painful.)

At the same time breathing is *quickened* so that sufficient oxygenation is obtained.

I advise women to use, when they refer to this type of breathing, the words *shallow* and *quickened*, as these words are associated with the reasons behind their action. They should not use the word *panting*, which is vague and does not suggest any reason for this type of breathing.

(*b*) Relaxation of the abdominal muscles so as to avoid side-to-side pressure on the uterus.

(*c*) Relaxation of the pelvic floor so as to avoid vertical compression at the level of the cervix and the inferior uterine segment.

(*d*) Relaxation of the muscles of the shoulder, back and buttocks.

Shallow and quickened breathing start to have effect from the time dilatation has reached the size of a quarter.

Muscular relaxation has a use from start to finish of labour, during contractions. From the time dilatation has reached the size of a quarter, until the end, it should be adhered to between contractions as well.

Three points have to be carefully kept in mind in this lecture:

Point 1. The shallow and quickened breathing, as well as relaxation, must *coincide* exactly with the physical signs preceding a contraction.

The woman must seek to ascertain these signs early in labour with the help of her assistant. During the period of dilatation to the size of a quarter they are:

(*a*) Movements somewhere in the uterus.

(*b*) More rarely movements of the child.

(*c*) Slight acceleration of the heart's rhythm over a very short time.

There is a fourth sign, which is not a physical one. This is the regular way in which the intervals between contractions get shorter and shorter, and takes the shape of a conditioned stimulus.

If the woman cannot spot these signs, she must seek assistance—this is what assistants are there for.

Point 2. The rupture of membranes is accompanied by loss of the waters. If it occurs at the beginning, one does not notice that it has any important effect on the contractions, be it their intensity or their frequency.

As a rule rupture takes place at a " quarter " dilatation, and is caused by contractions.

If no rupture takes place, this has to be done *artificially*, but it is a painless intervention. What must be kept in mind is this: be the rupture spontaneous or artificial, the head of the child will press more on the cervix and the contractions will be more intense and frequent. There will follow for the woman a more delicate moment of adaptation. She must become more attentive and respond still more to contractions as soon as they appear.

Point 3. As dilatation reaches its maximum, *contractions alter in quality and the woman's behaviour will at the same time alter in quality.* What held good until then holds good no longer; all the exits are wide open and all obstructions have been removed. Contractions have no longer the task of opening the cervix (this has been done); theirs is to push out the contents of the uterus—the child.

An inborn reflex based on the uterus comes into effect; an earnest request is thrust upon the woman. The phase of delivery has started, there is a wish to push, nay, a need to push.

Usually the need is discreet to start with, but it asserts itself with each new contraction until it has become well defined.

Sometimes the need to push comes on ruthlessly; attention must be drawn to it so as to avoid any loss of control that such a surprise would inevitably entail.

What the woman must know above all is that at such a moment she must warn the medical attendant or the midwife.

An examination is made, followed by a decision, in conformity with what she has been taught.

EXERCISES

Shallow and quickened breathing, plus muscular relaxation.

This is carried out at six different times of the day, one each time, in the following manner:

For thirty seconds at first, for two days.

Then thirty-five seconds for another two days.

Then forty seconds, sixty seconds, etc.

The lungs should be neither too filled nor too emptied. Breathing can be either through the mouth or the nose.

Respiratory exchanges should be equal.
Be modest to start with.
Do not try to breathe either too shallowly or too quickly.
The shoulders must not be shrugged.

Position: Lying down.
Flat on the back.
At times on one side.
At times sitting up.

LECTURE VI

THE DELIVERY

MANY women confusedly take labour to mean the stage of delivery; or, if you like, labour means delivery. Others look upon delivery as the climax of many hours of suffering.

We can say in no uncertain way today that we have found this to account for the major part of the apprehension and fear that women had of labour.

In fact, to them it all boiled down to a real *physical conflict*. A physical conflict in the sense that there appeared to exist an enormous difference of proportion. What I mean is the *difference between the size of the child and the dimensions of the birth canal*.

It is clear that in the light of their early education this set a distressing problem.

Nowadays the situation is very far from this. They know that delivery cannot take place without some initiatory processes. When we speak of initiatory processes, we mean not only all the organic and functional changes themselves (as shown in the preceding lecture), but also their operation during labour.

When they reach delivery they will know—they know it already—that no physical conflict exists; the disproportion between the size of the child and the dimensions of the birth canal evens itself out steadily as dilatation progresses. Obstacles disappear while tissues become softer and can respond, by stretching without difficulty, to any demand made by the advancing head of the child.

They will, therefore, participate in the most interesting stage of their labour in full possession of their faculties. It will be also the most active stage, and the one in which they will have to make the greatest effort.

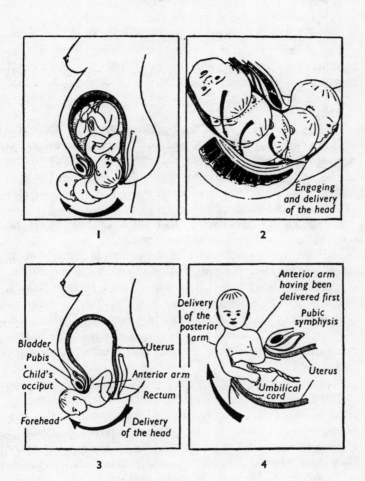

Figure 10

We shall remind them that delivery is characterised at its beginning by a wish, and by a *need to push*, which is an essential help to the uterus in expelling the child.

The quality of the contraction having changed, the woman's behaviour too will change in character. A rational response to the needs of delivery will demand that she realises several things.

They are:

1. The exact place and the precise position of the child in her abdomen, so that she should know where the expelling forces act. These act chiefly on the fundus of the uterus, and less so on its side walls. The resultant of these forces is in the direction of the exit—namely, the vaginal cavity and its vulvar opening.

2. The right time at which to push, this being when the contraction reaches its maximum intensity.

3. That it is a great mistake to push as if " straining at stools "; this should never be done. When the muscles of the pelvic floor contract they squeeze the rectum; this is fine when we are dealing with the physiology of defaecation, but they squeeze the vagina just as much. So if straining is indulged in it will obstruct the passage of the baby's head through the vagina. Hence it is an effort that is not called for.

4. The right way to push.

The diaphragm and the abdominal muscles are powerful friends of the contracting uterus. In the case of the diaphragm its downward descent during inspiration is used as a force pressing down on the fundus of the uterus. *More than that*, when the diaphragm has reached its lowermost position, by holding it there the abdominal muscles will get from the immobilised ribs *a solid and static purchase*. To ensure this indispensable purchase, one must inspire deeply and then hold this inspired air in one's lungs—that is, hold one's breath. The abdominal muscles are then brought into action; their upper part moves inwards and the force exerted by them must likewise act on the fundus of the uterus and must be directed towards the vaginal outlet.

To achieve this, the woman will have (after a first inspiration and expiration) to breathe in again and to hold her breath; then she touches her chest with her chin and keeps it there, followed by rounding her shoulders forwards and downwards—the bust being kept slightly flexed in the meantime. She will use her hands and arms to help her maintain this position.

5. The meaning of delivery—what must be done and, above all, what must not be done.

With each effort the parturient will feel the downward progress of the head in the pelvis. The wish to push will increase with each contraction and soon the child will be born.

Then, at the very moment when a new effort would disengage the head, the woman receives a bewildering order: " Stop pushing, please! "

To stop pushing she will have to start breathing rapidly; by so doing the diaphragm is *mobilised* and the abdominal muscles lose their purchase on the ribs. Without this bearing point they cannot work efficiently.

There follows then a short stage of delivery. By retaining full consciousness during it the woman will find her efforts fully rewarded. She will have worked to create life; she will have helped her child into this world, and it will not be a question of the child being laid into her arms after someone else has helped it into this world.

EXERCISES

The action of the muscles of the pelvic floor must be differentiated from that of the abdominal muscles during delivery. This is achieved by carrying out the following exercises:

1. Breathe in; hold your breath and try to strain as in defaecation.

2. Breathe in; hold your breath and try to pass water (micturate).

Do not carry out these two exercises from a purely mechanical point of view. Try to analyse them and see what takes place at the level of the pelvic floor.

During straining *the muscular effort* will be felt in a backwards and downwards direction; that is, towards the rectum.

During micturltion *the muscular effort* will be felt forwards and downwards, that is, towards the bladder.

During those two efforts the abdominal muscles are contracted. Their duty is to hold in position the abdominal contents; they do not move, working in a *static manner*.

But during delivery, when pressure is being exerted by the abdominal muscles, there is an inward movement of its upper portion; hence the difference between the two effects achieved must be differentiated in terms of the effort expanded. Once this differentiation has been appreciated, it is easier to use these muscles in a rational manner during labour.

If I ask for a repetition of the act of defaecation and of micturition, it is to make sure that a woman can keep the muscles of her pelvic floor in a relaxed state during delivery. These muscles can be trained like any other muscle.

These exercises should be carried out twice daily, at the same time that the relaxation exercises are practised (same principle).

The exercise of the effort of delivery is practised vigorously once a week, but *gently* twice daily. None of the exercises should be practised without medical advice.

THE PART PLAYED BY THE BRAIN

THIS lecture is devoted to an explanation of the mechanism of the brain; that is, the working of the brain. It is a very important lecture; in grasping how your brain works, you will understand how your activities will lead you to a labour without pain.

Your attention has been drawn in previous lectures to the important place occupied by the nervous system in our body. Since the brain is the principal part of the nervous system, it is, therefore, the directing organ of our body.

In the previous lectures you have been taught theoretical and practical things. As far as the theoretical ones go, it is clear that your brain has been responsible for recording them. It can be said that the same holds for the practical lessons you have been taught. In fact, when you practise the shallow and quickened breathing as during dilatation, or even the guided push as during delivery, you have the impression that only muscles have been called into play; true enough, there is certainly muscular activity, but the working of these muscles corresponds to the way in which the brain is functioning. It is precisely because your brain functions in a certain manner at the very moment your muscles are working that your activities will lead you to a labour without pain.

This lecture on the brain will, therefore, be divided into three parts:

1. The brain as the controlling organ of the body.
2. The functioning of the brain generally.
3. The functioning of the brain during painless childbirth.

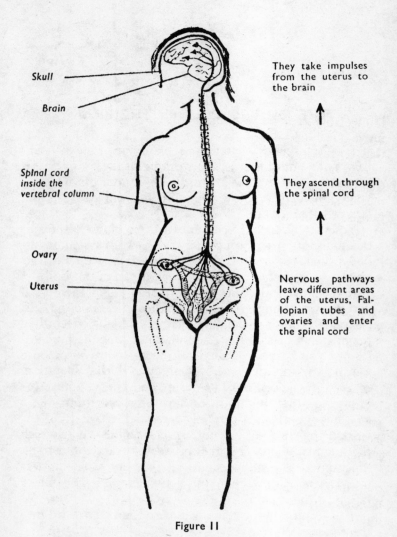

Skull

Brain

Spinal cord
inside the
vertebral column

Ovary

Uterus

They take impulses
from the uterus to
the brain

↑

They ascend through
the spinal cord

↑

Nervous pathways
leave different areas
of the uterus, Fal-
lopian tubes and
ovaries and enter
the spinal cord

Figure II

*It is in the brain that sensations are synthetised from
impulses coming from the uterus. The prevailing state of
the brain at that time will dictate the nature of the effect
such impulses cause*

1. THE BRAIN AS THE CONTROLLING ORGAN OF THE BODY

Nothing in the body escapes the control of the brain. We know, from long ago, that mobility—that is, the power to move our limbs—depends on brain function; we know too that sensitivity, which allows us to feel warm, cold, softness or hardness, equally depends on its function. Proof of this is to be found in lesions of the brain, when a hemiplegia may result; there is paralysis or even anaesthesia—that is, absence of sensory perception in some parts of the body.

We know too that our organs of special sense depend on the brain; especially the two most important ones—the eye and the ear. Our ears supply us with a sense of hearing, which means that we receive information about the world around us by means of sounds. Above all, our ears convey to the brain the special sounds made by the spoken word. Speech is nothing less than a succession of sounds with a meaning, and it is by means of these spoken words that fellow-men impart their thoughts to us.

In a similar way the eyes are responsible for vision. That is, we receive information about the world around us by means of images, movements, colours, shapes, etc., as well as by the written word. By means of writing our environment imparts its thoughts to us.

Finally, we know, thanks to the work of Pavlov, that our brain keeps under its dominance the functioning of our internal organs, such as the heart, lungs, kidneys, spleen, intestines, uterus, etc.

Our body in its entirety communicates with the brain through a complex network of nerves, the majority of which converge to form a special nervous strand called the " spinal cord " (Figure 11). This spinal cord lies in the spinal canal, which is within the vertebral column, formed by vertebra piled up one on top of the other. In a similar way the eyes communicate with the brain via the optic nerves, and the ears via the auditory nerves.

The brain receives "information" about the working of our various organs via this aggregate of nerves, and sends back its "orders" by the same system. It is the perpetual coming and going of information and orders, springing from the activity of the brain, which gives life to our body.

Now we have noticed that elements apparently unrelated to one another can come together within the brain; these elements bring, for example, information derived from our internal organs, or information passed on by our organs of special sense.

If we agree that it is by virtue of information received from our organs of sense that we formulate our thoughts, our cognition, etc., we soon see how these thoughts can act on and interfere with the working of our internal organs. To understand this we must study more intimately the working of the brain.

2. THE INTIMATE WORKING OF THE BRAIN

In the diagram (Figure 11) we see a profile of our brain, and we shall try, using a simple example, to imagine what goes on inside it. Let us consider the act of holding an object, a ruler, say. When we pick up the object we do so with an aim. We want this movement to have some effect. This movement has a certain effect because it is a harmonising one, and the various muscles which come into use work in perfect co-ordination. How does this come about? I can say that the moment I pick up an object or I lift a ruler it corresponds to something particular in my brain. This something is the creation of what is called a " focus of activity ". A focus of activity is the result of the combined functioning of a certain number of cortical cells. Now, when a focus of activity is engendered in some part of the brain, this focus has a tendency to develop and spread; that is, it irradiates.

Let us assume for one moment that this focus, brought about by the movement I made, develops and spreads. Well, instead of carrying out the simple movement consisting in lifting the ruler, I shall end by making disorganised gesticulations, contortions or going into convulsions; that is, the irradiation of this motor focus would fire off the whole motor activity of the brain.

To obtain the precise movement which I wish to carry out it is essential that the focus activated in some part of my brain remains localised and that this tendency to irradiation be forestalled. This is exactly what happens through a property of the brain which sees to the restriction of any development of this focus. In fact, as soon as a focus is created, that area of the brain around it reacts to it by an inverse phenomenon which opposes its development, " braking " it, so to speak. This braking property is called inhibition. This inhibition is, therefore, that zone in the brain which puts a stop to the spread of a focus of activity by refusing to function. Let us take a few simple examples to demonstrate the importance of this question of inhibition.

An easy example is that of a railway passenger who, lost in his novel, does not hear or hears indistinctly the conversations of the other passengers. What is going on in his brain?

Well, his reading activity corresponds to a cortical focus of activity. This focus is surrounded by a zone of inhibition which the excitations produced by the chit-chat of his neighbours reach. Since they have converged on this zone of inhibition, these excitations are not recorded and, therefore, the reader does not hear the conversations of the people around him.

In the same way, a pupil paying attention to his teacher's lecture is not aware of noises in the street because the attention he is paying to the lecture corresponds to a focus of activity in his brain, and this focus becomes surrounded by a zone of inhibition into which all the stimuli from the surrounding noises drain.

Let us take the opposite example. The pupil does not follow the lecture and is listening to the street noises. We say that he is absent-minded. What goes on in his brain? In the same way, when he listens to the street noises this corresponds to a focus of activity surrounded by a zone of inhibition which the teacher's words reach, and which are thus not recorded.

Let us take a third, still more interesting, example. We have all at some time or another suffered from toothache. We have noticed how the pain could fluctuate; easily bearable, even unnoticed, as we were busily lost in some important occupation; stabbing as we brood over nothing through inactivity. In the first instance our occupation corresponds to a cerebral focus of activity which becomes surrounded by a zone of inhibition into which the stimuli coming from the diseased tooth reach. Ending in this zone, they are poorly registered, if at all. Conversely, during inactivity only the focus produced by the diseased tooth is active, and this focus has all the room it wants to spread.

We can see from these examples how important inhibition is. It is this braking phenomenon which allows the brain to choose a certain function, and to favour one at the expense of another. It is, above all, important to understand how this inhibition works with regard to the working of our internal organs (and we shall see soon how this takes place with regard to the uterus). It is important to understand how this inhibition comes about, because it is precisely on its application that the whole preparation to childbirth without pain is based.

Let us take, as a simple case, the working of our stomach. During digestion the stomach works in two ways: food is chemically altered by the gastric juices, while they are synchronously altered physically by the contractions of the gastric musculature. This double action constitutes digestion as it is at each of our meals. Now when the stomach contracts it irritates nerve endings; this gives rise to a stimulus that goes to the brain. By and large, we do not happen to feel this gastric contraction; that is, this stimulus is not registered. Why is it not registered? Because the many, the very many, activities we undertake in a day give rise to as many foci of activity; and they, by inducing zones of inhibition, halt the entry of stimuli caused by the contraction of the gastric muscles.

However, there are times when we are aware of this contraction, in the form of the type called " gastric cramp ". What are the circumstances in which stimuli are thus registered by the brain? Such circumstances, we have noticed, as those in which we are subject to an extremely powerful emotion, like fear, for example. Following intense fear, we feel completely exhausted, shaking, " whacked out ", as we say. The exhaustion which we feel corresponds to a sudden lowering of the activity potential of our brain; the intense emotion exacts from our brain a sudden discharge of energy, and the latter finds itself completely drained out soon after. In such a case the cerebral potential is lowered as a whole, the positive activity at par with inhibition is correspondingly diminished. Inhibition, provisionally diminished, is not strong enough to oppose the entrance of gastric stimulation in the brain. It is then that it becomes registered and makes itself felt as a gastric cramp.

The same thing is true for what we call " palpitations", which are felt during some intense upset. These cardiac palpitations correspond to the recording by the brain of the contraction of the heart muscle, which normally gives rise to stimuli held in abeyance by the braking system of the cortex.

We therefore see that it is this inhibition activity which decides whether the brain will register excitations coming from internal organs and, by this means, the function of these organs may or may not be perceived. We shall see that it is the very same phenomenon which acts during labour.

3. The Working of the Brain during Labour

Strictly speaking, childbirth is brought about by the contraction of the uterine muscle; it can be said that labour is nothing else but the sum of uterine contractions. In the first instance they lead to dilatation; in the second instance they lead to delivery. These uterine contractions are felt in a definite way which, when very intense, gives rise to pain.

Why are these contractions felt? Because the nervous stimulation produced by them is registered by the brain. Why should the brain register it? Because the latter cannot hold the pain back by sufficient inhibition. Why, then, should this inhibition prove inadequate? As a whole, the brain of the pregnant woman, by virtue of her ignorance, is the prey of small emotional upsets repeated thousands of times and linked with fear and apprehension of childbirth. It is as if it were in a state of inferiority, being more so at the very time of childbirth, when fear becomes accentuated and the activity potential is in consequence further lowered. Its activity potential having thus foundered, the brain cannot build up an inhibition powerful enough to oppose the intrusion of the nervous stimulation produced by uterine contraction. Thus registered, uterine contraction produces pain; this pain in turn lowers further the activity potential of the brain, diminishing still further the latter's power of inhibition, and thereby creates a vicious circle.

How can this vicious circle be broken? How can one stop the uterine impulses from getting through? By reinforcing the inhibition of the brain. This is exactly it, and the aim of all the preparation that has been given is to reinforce to its maximum the inhibition of the brain. The problem is to know how to achieve maximum effective inhibition.

We saw, when we started, that inhibition was always produced by the presence of a focus of activity. It can be said that at the very moment a pregnant woman is told of the existence of childbirth without pain a focus of activity starts in her mind. As her preparation progresses and gains ground, so this focus extends and becomes reinforced. In fact, all types of occupation, be they intellectual or physical, correspond to a focus of activity. The physical exercises that you are taught help towards reinforcing this focus and, above all, promote its spread during labour itself. In fact, the focus of activity engendered by a preparation exhibits itself only during labour, since at any other time the brain is busy with a horde of other activities. Your preparation, as well as the training you are undergoing, consists in educating your brain to channel all its potential force into one, and only one, focus of activity, namely, that which corresponds to your labour.

It is just the attention with which you will follow your labour, and with which you will apply the exercises you have learnt, that will develop the focus of activity necessary for the creation of effective inhibition. And the more powerful this focus the more effective and able will the inhibition be in stopping the effect of uterine impulses. I must stress the fact that the intensity of that focus will depend mostly on the intensity of the effort displayed by you during your labour; and the ease with which this focus will come to life depends equally on the work and training which you will have yourselves done.

This is most important, because it means that the strength of the inhibition depends on the strength of the focus, and the strength of that focus depends on the effort contributed by you; hence the success of your labour is entirely in your hands. The success of labour is a direct variant of the woman's own contribution.

To sum up, it is a question of creating in the brain a focus of activity for the purpose of generating an inhibiting effect which will resist the development of a cerebral focus initiated by nervous stimuli from uterine contractions. This is done through a knowledge of the phenomena that appear during labour as well as by practising some exercises, such as shallow and quickened breathing, or guided push.

The training undertaken by the woman, the work she puts in on her own account, amounts in fact to training the brain to establish this focus of activity in such a way that during a labour the watchful attention of the woman, as well as her active awareness, will cause this focus to surge out with activity.

Thus it is exactly in this sense that the woman rules her labour. This question of active awareness on the part of the woman is an important question, as is her training which, when it comes to it, is instrumental in creating the focus of activity that serves as the starting point of the essential inhibition.

To conclude, we shall say that if the preparation consists of the *woman's rehearsal of her attitude during pregnancy* this will have two sequels. Firstly, the question of " believing " or " not believing " in painless childbirth does not arise; it is a question of rational education, not of " belief ". Secondly, since it is a question of learning how to give birth to a child, it is not a matter of " will " that abolishes pain, but *knowing* how to do it.

Finally, many women describing themselves as " nervous " fear that this " nervousness " may handicap them. In fact, what is commonly called nervousness is a state of the brain in which its activity is being exhibited in a chaotic and disorganised way. Training for childbirth is precisely learning how to *put this activity of the brain to use* in a rational manner. Hence the better prepared you are, the better will you use this activity—that is, your " nervousness " will be on your side. Contrariwise, it will act against you if your preparation is inadequate.

So, you are back on the school benches; be " good students " and you will reap the great and just reward of bringing your child into this world in a state of happiness.

FINAL LECTURE

FOR a long time we made the mistake of looking upon this lecture as a revision course.

It was a mistake because many women felt that there was no need to go over what they thought they had grasped perfectly well. This revision was therefore superfluous.

We are not completely in agreement with this point of view. On the contrary, we feel that every means should be used to anchor all these principles and all these new conceptions more firmly in one's mind. And they are far from easy.

We were also mistaken because we had more to say, and because there was a need for a reclassification.

This final focusing must be carried out without turning it into an *enumeration* of all the physical methods that make delivery painless. There are no physical methods which on their own can bring about this miracle, no more than one would say that painless childbirth was the result of cerebral action only.

We shall go over the various ways in which the start of labour presents itself:

1. *Commonest way.* This is marked by the appearance of contractions coming on at shorter and shorter regular intervals as labour progresses. The intensity of these regular contractions increases.
2. *Second way.* Loss of blood and mucous plug. If regular contractions accompany these signs, labour has started.
3. *Third way.* The breaking of the membranes, with the loss of waters.

When a woman has observed these signs what should

she do? When must she report to the obstetric hospital, should she be booked there?

Let us say straight away that the biggest mistake one could make *now* would be to advise her to *wait*. Wait for what *reasons*?

Because it is a question of prophylaxis, and Pavlov has shown us how the many excitations emanating from the external environment exert their influence on the subject.

A woman who has regularly attended her preparation course has accumulated a solid knowledge of the physiology of pregnancy and labour. We have strong doubts about the well-founded knowledge that would be possessed by her intimate circle or, more widely, her social circle. We do not mean by this that the woman lives in an inadequate environment; but the influence that such a circle could exert on her must take first place in our concern for her.

We cannot afford to leave it to chance.

We hope that in the not too distant future this risk will have disappeared.

However, any preparation for childbirth has been, is, and will remain the business of people qualified professionally to carry out its development, its teaching and its application. Childbirth must stay under medical supervision.

But maternity interests everybody because it is a social phenomenon. When every one of us is familiar with the essential problems set by childbirth, when everyone is in a position to play his own part in resolving these problems, then pain in childbirth will be a thing of the past, once conceived and nurtured by society.

We are not there yet.

We therefore advise every woman not to wait once the contractions have started.

It is far better for her to reach the obstetric hospital too soon than too late. It is much better that she should come in, even if nothing happens. In such a case, a chat with her will show errors of interpretation or gaps in her knowledge that will explain precisely why she reported to hospital without justification.

The woman should, as soon as the first signs of labour present themselves, carry out a complete revision of what she has been taught.

Not to wait does not imply that she must rush.

She must meet the first five or six contractions by complete muscular relaxation as well as a shallow and quickened respiration; but above all she should study the way these contractions behave. This includes their starting point, their intensity, the alteration in the shape of the uterus, the way these contractions regress before disappearing and, finally, the reason for their presence.

The response to the first contractions is specially important in the multiparous. She will prove to herself that these *contractions are normally perceptible* and that they have nothing in common with the *pains* of her previous deliveries. These realities will blot out past memories.

The future mother should, before the expected date of her confinement, have ready all the necessary things and papers that she has to take with her. She should also foresee what means of transport she can fall back on, should she require them. Nothing should be left to chance. The best time to leave her home is at the end of a contraction.

Between leaving home and reaching the hospital, each time she feels a contraction she should practise shallow and quickened breathing, while relaxing as best she can.

At the first examination in hospital, dilatation is usually found to have hardly progressed. At this early stage of labour all unjustified expenditure of energy should be avoided. Usually, primigravidas are advised to sleep, but note that the parturient may then be woken up by a strong contraction. All she need do then is to take a few deep breaths and come out of her slumbers (thus heightening the threshold of cortical perception). At the next contraction no painful sensation is discerned. Other primigravidas will find that reading or writing is a useful pastime.

Multiparous women find it in their interest to keep a watch on their old associations so that they should not gain a footing.

After dilatation has reached the size of a quarter the drill is the same for everybody. Once more we go over this and mention again that the evacuation of the placenta means complete delivery.

After this we proceed to go over every separate exercise taught. It is here that we must carefully ensure that they are linked with the reasons that justify them. We do our utmost to see that no woman completes her preparation with the thought that just by knowing " how to relax " she will have a painless labour; or that by knowing " how to breathe " she will have a painless confinement.

The preparation for painless childbirth is the interplay of many factors, both theoretical and practical, closely linked with one another. Any one factor on its own has no meaning and no effect.

After repeating the exercises, the patients are taken round the maternity wards and the labour wards, so that they can become acquainted with the place of their confinement. We end by introducing them to recently-delivered women. There follows much questioning and much answering. It is most useful to bring these women face to face, because it serves to confirm the value of their training. No better confirmation could be given than that of a woman who has proved it for herself.

PART IV

NECESSARY CONDITIONS FOR THE REALISATION OF CHILDBIRTH WITHOUT PAIN

CHAPTER I

PRACTICAL CONDITIONS

IT will be useful to give some precise facts on the conditions necessary for the psychoprophylactic preparation for painless childbirth.

One of the objections to this method has been said to be the fact that it required important facilities which were practically unobtainable under the present circumstances.

Childbirth without pain was in fact a fine ideal, but impossible to reach as it was very complicated and costly.

These criticisms do not hold water.

Painless childbirth is a fact. Thousands of women in France and neighbouring countries will vouch for it. It has already been obtained under varying conditions—in public hospitals, in private nursing homes, by doctors and midwives in private practice, and even in rural districts with poor means of transport. Everywhere similar results have been obtained when the psychoprophylactic method has been applied strictly according to set technique.

Indeed, the psychoprophylactic method, if founded on the complex laws relating to higher nervous activity, is simple and precise in its technical realisation. It stands in sharp contrast here to some methods relying on drugs which can be applied only in a hospital centre equipped specially for them.

Its realisation demands two conditions:

(a) A thorough preparation given by qualified people.
(b) A guarantee of peace, silence, comfort and the help of a qualified assistant during the whole of the labour.

1. MATERIAL AND FACILITIES REQUIRED

(A) PREPARATION

The material required consists of charts showing the various stages of pregnancy and labour, and of a film at the end of the course of preparation.

It is important that the preparation should take place in a special room where the women feel at home, and in pleasant surroundings which will make them attentive and encourage them to ask questions.

(B) LABOUR

In hospital, the following conditions should be aimed at:

1. Separate labour wards allowing each parturient to be on her own, not hindered by the presence of neighbours.

It is equally necessary to try and have separate wards for the delivery of women who for some reason or other have not followed the course, or whose labour is not taking place under good conditions.

2. Near each labour bed there should be a supply of oxygen ready for inhalation.

3. Comfort given by firm rubber mattresses, and pillows or cushions in sufficient numbers. This is suggested if complete neuromuscular relaxation is to be encouraged.

4. Indirect lighting during labour so as to avoid tiring the eyes of the parturient.

5. Side light during the stage of delivery.

2. STAFF

This is the essential pillar on which the success of childbirth without pain rests.

It is imperative to have an educated staff, whatever its status.

Any person intimately or remotely concerned with the unit working towards painless childbirth must be educated, as this person will affect the parturients. Each person plays a part in creating the atmosphere, the tone that must prevail in the Maternity Unit. The four essential qualities are:

1. Gentle behaviour and voice.
2. Kindness of action.
3. Understanding, which always brings one nearer the woman.
4. Calmness, which does away with impatience.

These qualities must be possessed by the medical and para-medical staff as well as by the administrative or official staff.

The choice of such a staff demands a specially careful selector.

First of all, the staff as a whole should be re-educated. Each person is informed about the method, its essential principles and the practical conditions for its proper running. By means of a reasoned explanation, all those concerned become convinced that such a method can be applied. Each person is shown how, in her job, she is instrumental in bringing success by watching her attitude, her bearing, her actions and her words. Every woman who walks into the Maternity Unit must feel she is surrounded by friends who are eager to bear with her and help her.

Everything must create an impression of ease and security. The parturient must not feel the need to fall back on herself or be on the defensive.

A much more thorough briefing must, in time, be given to the nurses and midwives who will help the woman during labour. This personnel should know the technique of psychoprophylactic labour thoroughly. This demands that they should have at least an elementary understanding of the principles of higher nervous activity on which the method is founded.

They should also learn how to behave with discipline. Childbirth without pain is attained above all by team-work. Each case, above all each failure, should be studied and discussed together, and advantage taken of this to enhance the knowledge of the staff.

Valuable information here can be obtained from reports made by delivered women. They allow the staff to see, precisely, in each case, the consequences of an error or an act of negligence.

The collective work must be constantly reviewed and improved. Nothing must be left to chance in childbirth without pain; here, more than anywhere else, red tape is the number one enemy. Everyone, from the highest to the lowest, must be convinced of the necessity for constant improvement.

As far as the necessary number of staff goes, the object is that in the labour ward each parturient should be helped, right through labour, by a qualified person—doctor, midwife or specially trained nurse.

The setting up of all these conditions calls for additional expenses, which at the moment amount to four or five thousand francs per delivery; 90 per cent of this sum is spent on additional staff, both for the preparation and the bedside attendance. In some cases these additional expenses have been partly met by the *Sécurité Sociale.*

A circular from the *Ministère du Travail* has authorised the local treasuries of the *Sécurité Sociale* to raise (within the ceiling fixed for the nearest public centre dealing with the same problems) the daily expenses of recognised maternity units where painless childbirth by the psychoprophylactic method has been in force.

This participating interest is unfortunately limited at the moment only to recognised clinics, because the national commission on the nomenclature of medical Acts of the *Sécurité Sociale* has not yet secured approval to include the psychoprophylactic method for painless childbirth in the nomenclature.

It is fervently hoped that this participation may be extended. Painless childbirth should be a matter for the State.

It is fairly clear even from a purely financial point of view, leaving aside the enormous social and humane advantages, that painless childbirth offers to the public in general a good investment.

Its short-term advantages include a reduction in the time spent in hospital after delivery, an important reduction in the use of drugs, a reduction in the number of obstetric interventions.

It also has long-term advantages which are difficult to show in figures, but nevertheless considerable.

A bill has been lodged with the office of the *Assemblée Nationale* implying that the financial responsibility for the additional expenses of the psychoprophylactic method should come from the budget for *Santé Publique*. Let us hope that such a project is achieved in this way or some other.

While waiting for the method to be adopted on a nation-wide basis, we hope that local authorities—municipal or regional—will follow the example set by the Municipal Council of Paris, which voted, for the year 1954, the sum of fifteen million francs towards the realisation of the psychoprophylactic method in six maternity units of the Public Assistance.

This sum was raised to thirty-five million for 1955.

We further hope that the Treasury of the *Sécurité Sociale*, within its social and health framework, will add the weight of its financial support to the extension of the practice of childbirth without pain.

CHAPTER II

GENERAL CONDITIONS

CHILDBIRTH without pain gives constant figures of its true results only when it is applied in " total unison ". This will be when women, public services and medical bodies join forces for its general application under the best possible conditions. As events make this still far from reality, those women who have earned the trust of sincere pioneers hold in their hands the reins of success and will know how to tower over any petty obstacles and come through triumphant.

It seems to us imperative that women should be aware of the irregular results obtained by some applications of the method.

This is due to several reasons:

(*a*) Some experimenters talk of childbirth without pain when they apply some mongrel method which has nothing to do with the psychoprophylactic approach. Each method certainly has its good points, but should not be mistaken for or likened to any other method. " Childbirth Without Fear ", " Natural Childbirth ", " Psychosomatic Childbirth " are methods which have been clearly described by their authors, but they differ from the psychoprophylactic method both in theory and in practice, as shown in previous chapters.

(*b*) By using the same names confusion between methods that have different preparations is deliberately created, and then people seek to compare the results obtained.

In order to draw an honest comparison of results, the same method must be followed with the same scientific discipline and under the same experimental conditions, and the same objective spirit must pervade it. A method which prepares women in nine sessions is different from one which prepares them in 15 or 20 or more sessions. A method which emphasises exercises and one which stresses the essential role of education cannot claim to have the same principles.

(c) Some experimenters systematically administer a whiff of gas at the end of delivery, or as the child is being delivered. They feel, so they say, that this cuts out the trying and painful sensation following the stretching of the perineum. This attitude finds no place in painless childbirth. The woman who has striven for hours to control and direct her labour will not suffer the exhilarating moment she longs for and which she awaits intensively, the moment when, seeing her child come into the world, she will have achieved a wonderful purpose, to be stolen from her. It is a breach of trust and a mark of complacency on the part of the obstetrician. Anaesthesia should be used only in cases reckoned by the obstetrician or midwife to be difficult. Those who still maintain that anaesthesia should be used during delivery can never have seen the face of a woman who has herself brought her child into the world.

No obstetrician or midwife can forget that face, radiant with joy and full of pride, as the mother sees her child being born. Once she has experienced this she does not want to be delivered in any other way.

(d) By creating doubt, by voluntarily nurturing confusion, one delays the evolution and application of a method that sweeps away our old beliefs and opens the door for a more humanitarian approach.

We are, therefore, called upon to expound the essential factors on which painless childbirth and its success depend.

Four factors come into play in different degrees. We shall classify them in what appears to us their order of importance:

1. The material conditions, about which we shall say little, since they have been dealt with in the preceding chapter.
2. The future mother herself.
3. The administrative and ancillary staff.
4. The medical staff: obstetrician, physician and midwife.

1. Material Conditions

We would like to add something about the material conditions. If they have to be changed in order to change the conditions of labour themselves, they must not become an alibi for not practising childbirth without pain. We hear very frequently arguments such as: " We would like to apply the method as it is a good one, but it is too costly. . . . Many alterations must be made in clinics, and the preparation is an expensive one." All these arguments do not hold for one moment. Little is needed, and only few expenses, to change the atmosphere in a labour ward—a cheerful painting, some flowers, some nice photographs and, above all, a welcoming atmosphere created by a charming, friendly and understanding staff. Quiet need no longer be requested; it occurs naturally as women cease to scream and the staff goes about calmly and silently. The material conditions for the realisation of the method will be perfected in stages, in keeping with the progress of the method itself.

As far as the preparation goes, this will depend only on the social services (subsidies by municipalities to maternity centres, increase in lump sums, etc., by the *Sécurité Sociale*) and, therefore, does not lead to any additional expenses for the women.

Childbirth without pain must not and should not be the prerogative of well-to-do classes only. Women, regardless of their status in society, must be granted the privilege of bringing their children into the world without pain.

2. THE FUTURE MOTHER HERSELF

The most unfavourable factor at the moment is the doubt that many try to create, or simply foster, in the minds of women.

A doubt fed and fanned by preceding generations which holds that it is impossible for a woman to go through labour without pain, or which minimises labour in asserting (as a reaction) that " there is nothing terrible about it and that one should not make a song and dance about it ". The fact is that before the growth of painless childbirth women always depicted labour as a trying experience, even if they had an easy time. It would be of great benefit if mothers encouraged their daughters to follow this training so that they could give birth to their children under excellent conditions and cherish one of the finest memories of their life. Proof of this is shown by the existence of families in which childbirth is easy; this is due to the fact that confinement is not depicted in dramatic terms, but as a normal event in the life of a woman. This attitude must be cultivated and it is the greatest gift that society can bestow on the future generations of mothers.

There is also a doubt in the mind of some medical people (who, however, are getting fewer and fewer) who, refusing to believe in the method, deny its existence. This attitude is very bad as the practitioner, who exerts considerable influence on his patients, may for a while hinder the progress of the method. There again, as the number of educated women increases, they will convince the wavering practitioners and ignore those who systematically oppose the method.

One would think that the woman who has favoured the psychoprophylactic method for her labour would remain immune from any influences once she has made the decision. This is not always the case, and from the very beginning she must be warned of the pitfalls by the following:

(*a*) *Her own education:* her school friends, her experience of life, the important milestones in her life as a woman, chiefly her first periods and her first intercourse.

(*b*) *Her family background:* this includes the circle in which she has grown up, her present circle, her husband's influence, and that of her parents-in-law.

(*c*) *Her circle:* her friends or her colleagues, whatever her social standing.

(*d*) *Her own make-up:* intellectual people (professors, doctors, and members of the liberal professions, etc.) have to face greater problems still. We have definitely observed that if a woman doctor, or a teacher, goes through the school of painless childbirth with the same modesty as the working woman she will have a successful, painless delivery. On the other hand, if she keeps her intellectual conceit, she is certain to fail.

(*e*) *Society as a whole*, which is poorly educated and holds on to its out-of-date principles which can only be shed with difficulty. A natural apathy and poor reading foster this attitude.

All these difficulties will disappear the day society as a whole adopts the right attitude towards this problem. This could be achieved in one generation, two at the most. Within three years China made rapid progress along those lines.

3. The Administrative and Ancillary Staff

We shall do no more than stress the great importance of ensuring their education, the aims and principles of which have been discussed in the preceding chapters.

4. The Medical Staff

As they play the most important part in the preparation and the confinement, they should possess a detailed knowledge of the theory, technique and practice of the method, thus avoiding serious mistakes and being themselves partially responsible for its failures. The medical staff should, therefore, also review their attitude and completely repudiate their good or bad habits, to reintegrate them within the framework of childbirth without pain, after having adapted them to the demands of such a practice. The essential and most difficult task will be to create their own conditioning, which includes:

1. The attitude towards the parturient during pregnancy and labour.
2. Medical changes in the choice of words, hence altering their own vocabulary.
3. Finding the enthusiasm and energy which must permeate the method.

This triumph over oneself entails a huge effort which will yield its maximum effect only in work done as a team.

Childbirth without pain must ensure the formation of teams of obstetricians and midwives, which will guarantee more rational and more valuable results and which will constantly improve relationships within the team and with the parturient. In childbirth without pain each contributor must give of his best.

CHAPTER III

APPLICATION OF THE METHOD

WE thought that it would be invaluable for colleagues and midwives to have precise information about our views on the present facilities for the practice of the method.

We shall pose four questions:

1. Can the method be applied (*a*) in country practice, (*b*) in domiciliary practice, (*c*) in a small maternity home, or is it strictly meant for specialised centres only?
2. Does the method apply to all obstetrical cases and to all women?
3. Has it any dangers?
4. What is required for its general application?

QUESTION 1

This method, whose value has now been confirmed by wide experience, can also be applied in special circumstances. This demands that it should be practised by a medical man well read in its physiological basis and well versed in its practice.

The Russians have shown that the method could be applied in country districts.

In small Chinese villages as far away from a big centre as 320, 500 or 650 miles, Chinese women can equally well be delivered amidst joy. This radical transformation was achieved essentially by the use of the most basic principle in the method: EDUCATION. These country practitioners have gone back to their books to study Pavlovian physiology and its application to obstetrics. They have relearnt their obstetrics in the light of the new conditions brought about by the application of such a method.

In France such a possibility exists, as has been shown by the initiative of a few practitioners.

A doctor of the *Sécurité Sociale* read to a gathering of the Association of Country Practitioners in a region of the South of France a paper entitled " The Country Doctor and Psychoprophylactic Childbirth ". He delivered a practical exposition of the method, and put in a simple way the contents of lectures or interviews to be given to the pregnant woman. If this example were followed in all regions, an important step would be taken towards the education of the medical world, and a change of its attitude towards this problem and to parturients.

Another example deserves mention here. It relates to the work of a married couple in a small village in south-west France. In this little village of a few hundred inhabitants, these two practitioners applied the method, working as a perfect team. How did they go about it ? They chose to be taught and to witness the results of the method. Having been convinced, they went back to their village bent on applying the method. Their experience was to be a thorough one, because the wife herself gave birth to a child painlessly. They started teaching a few women—no mean task when one is not trained as a teacher. The husband's education, and that of the woman's family circle, was carried out with patience. Soon the educational effort bore its fruits; the first woman who gave birth without pain spurred them on and made their task easier. The village spoke of nothing else but childbirth without pain, and a combined effort of human generosity sprang up! All newly delivered women became precious collaborators of the practitioner and any future mother. So education reduced the load on the individual practitioner, who then played his true part as a guiding force. Now every woman has her child at home, in a converted homely atmosphere, with everyone knowing what part to play. Husband, mother, mother-in-law or grandmother have all changed their way of talking. An era of understanding has displaced, with the impulse of the two doctors, an era of sterile and decadent routine.

Any country doctor, helped by his wife or by an instructed and convinced assistant, can also achieve this miracle which will bring to him unheard of and unqualified pleasure and satisfaction.

It is just as possible in a small maternity home. It will be simplified by the fact that the number of people to be educated is small. It will need a well-trained obstetrician and midwife to change the mental outlook of the staff, that is, alter the atmosphere of the clinic. The material atmosphere will follow suit. Quietness will result by the women themselves ceasing to scream; cheerfulness will spring from the happy faces of the delivered women and of the staff and with the gay presence of flowers.

A larger maternity centre (with problems of organisation as the result of a greater medical and ancillary staff) should act as a guiding centre in a district where a maternity school allows scattered doctors to come to see their successes and, above all, their failures. Each person learns something from the next; obstetrics will progress and the health of mother and child will improve. The practitioner himself will feel happier and more secure in his special work.

QUESTION 2

The preparation can be offered and should be offered without discrimination to every pregnant woman. As we have already said, this instruction is but a stage in the education that all young girls should be given during adolescence. This is why we feel that its general propagation is absolutely essential to the radical change in the mental outlook that a pregnant woman has towards her confinement, regardless of the method used.

As for the application of the method during labour, we

are in a position after four years of experience, to confirm that it is beneficial to women.

During the Congress of Obstetricians and Gynaecologists of the French-speaking world, held in Brussels in September 1955, we illustrated this opinion by a report on the use of the method in a few special obstetrical conditions, as in:

1. Pulmonary lesions.
2. Cardiac lesions.
3. Cases of breech presentation.
4. Abnormal presentation.

We have also demonstrated the possibility open to obstetricians in several proved cases, of using forceps (Suzor) without anaesthesia. Here are a few examples of this use:

1. To facilitate a painful rotation in posterior presentations.
2. To help the descent of the head where the pelvis has a low symphysis.
3. To deliver the child quickly in cases of foetal distress.
4. To help the descent of the head of a premature child or a very big child.
5. To help the descent of the head in cases with cardiac, pulmonary, asthmatic or hyperthyroid lesions.

We feel that it can be applied in all cases in which a long and difficult delivery is likely to tire the parturient. In these numerous special cases, the method, which after all is a physiological one, will spare the maximum expenditure of energy in the mother. She will reach the stage of delivery in a better state, and can expel her child without requiring inhalation of anaesthesia. This benefits the mother and, still more, the child.

Finally, in cases in which the obstetrician for some definite reason (abnormalities of the pelvis, extended head, short cord, etc.) after a trial of labour decides to do a

Caesarean section, this will be carried out under better conditions, for several reasons:

(*a*) The prepared woman will place herself completely in the hands of those who surround her, and the obstetrician's decision is accepted by her and her next of kin without discussion.

(*b*) The prepared woman undergoes calmly a length of trial labour and reaches Caesarean section in a good mental and physical state.

(*c*) The prepared woman, being calm and collected, will let the anaesthetist send her to sleep with a *greatly reduced* amount of anaesthesia. This will immediately be evident in mother and child.

All these interventions illustrate, furthermore, the point which we can never stress too often—that only the obstetrician can direct and regulate the progress of labour by such a method, the midwife dealing with normal cases and adding her assistance in all other cases.

We feel too that this method should not be kept for some women only. Any discrimination in a ward or in one's practice points to a shortcoming in the method. The woman who is excluded will look upon herself as abnormal and will worry during her pregnancy, reaching labour in an ill frame of mind. Having delivered women of all races, all colours, and under all conditions, we feel that any discrimination is a psychological error prejudicial to the woman. When the day comes when all women will have been prepared, as is the case in our practice, we shall be in a position to say that it is in the nature of the words used that the preparation may vary, depending on the intellectual status of the woman. Thus the manner of speech will be different if we are talking to a woman from the country, a city dweller, an illiterate woman or an intellectual one. One will always have to take the background of women into consideration. The physiological and scientific bases of the method are hard and fast, and the duty of education is to adapt them to the needs of the audience.

QUESTION 3

The greatest danger that may befall the method is that it should be badly applied as a result of being badly understood. It is not meant to be an easy method, and, therefore, it cannot be entrusted to any hands. It is a physiological and obstetrical method, and so demands a basic and sufficient knowledge of these two subjects. This is why we feel that obstetricians would be wrong to leave the preparation to ancillary staff not acquainted with the elementary principles of obstetrics. Physiotherapists and specialised nurses can become part of the team, but cannot pretend to educate women by themselves, replacing medical people and midwives. Nor must it be left completely in the hands of psychotherapists. They have a very definite place in the team as well as playing a precise part in educating the women; but the obstetrician is and must remain the *only head* in directing and controlling the preparation and the labour. As he is the only one conversant with the dynamic nature of the uterus, he alone can decide how such and such a labour is progressing.

The psychoprophylactic method, more than any other method applied in childbirth, demands a thorough knowledge of obstetrics. Hence, each case will be a new experience for the obstetrician and in each case he, more than anybody else, will know how to get the most out of the method. In no case, as some people are trying to affirm, will a prepared woman deliver herself painlessly without the advice of the obstetrician and the watchful care of the midwife. Team-work is an essential; it may be a team of two to start with which will later expand, but, as in all teams, there can only be one leader—and this is the obstetrician. Similarly, the training of midwives and ancillary staff, if it is to be thorough, must be undertaken by no one else but the obstetrician aware of his responsibilities. Otherwise, it will be easy to rob the method of its true structure and its educational value, and transform it into some nondescript monster. The results then will be poor and will fall prey to any counter-propaganda. But we feel that women, as they become warned, will not accept any malpractice or counterfeit. Childbirth without pain is for us all, both women and practitioners, a matter of conscience and honesty; no cheating can be allowed by one side or the other.

QUESTION 4

We saw that the U.S.S.R. and China have succeeded in spreading the method almost completely throughout their territory. We may wonder whether in other countries, such an extension is possible.

After several months of experience at various levels (hospitals, private clinics, countryside, etc.) we have come to the conclusion that this is possible.

To achieve this it is necessary that a few changes be made:

(*a*) A radical change in the conditions of confinement.

(*b*) A radical change in the plan of work of obstetricians and midwives.

(*c*) A change in the teaching of obstetrics in medical faculties and in the wards.

(A) CHANGE IN CONDITIONS OF CONFINEMENT

This amounts to asking for and obtaining funds from the *Santé Publique* in connection with the evolution of medical science and the ever-increasing needs of the public. This must result in a change for the better in antenatal clinics and a radical improvement in maternity wards, so that they lose their austere, inhuman and unsuitable atmosphere. They must cease to be frightening places; they must become places full of happiness and hope.

It is the duty of the *Sécurité Sociale*, which aims at seeing that everybody is properly looked after, to help this expanding work; and it will derive some profit in the long run, both for children and mothers—a fact that is not without weight. Prophylaxis is always less expensive than curative medicine.

(B) CHANGES IN THE PLAN OF WORK

Painless childbirth, as we have mentioned many times, means an additional effort on behalf of the medical profession. One must educate the women, one must educate the husbands and, before long, educate the children in those problems of life which must no longer be looked upon as belonging to the realms of mystery.

Childbirth itself demands more frequent visits and added efforts on the part of the medical adviser. This new enthusiastic task cannot be undertaken by one person alone. Some change in the plan of work of obstetricians must be formulated; teams have to be formed in which obstetricians and midwives join to produce a better output of work, both quantitatively and qualitatively, while remaining within human possibilities. There again it is a question of organisation, goodwill and economy.

In this organisation the midwife, whose standard is at present being continuously lowered, will find once more her true career as the close assistant and collaborator of the obstetrician.

Each group of people will thus be reinstated to its true status, which can but better the relationship between their various groups.

Hence there will no longer be a question of saying that this branch of medicine is overstaffed.

(C) CHANGES IN TEACHING

It is no intention of ours to change or upset teaching of undeniable value, but we feel that such teaching should include lectures on prophylaxis and more emphasis on physiology. Doctors and midwives come from faculties and Medical Schools. They must, therefore, from the start, be instructed in this new method which will later dictate their attitude towards the mothers of tomorrow. They must appreciate the role and importance of " wards ", so as to use them to the maximum good of everybody concerned.

It is only when future doctors and midwives have received such teaching that they will be able to impress, without effort or difficulty, the hospital staff under their control. More than that, by setting the example, they will create a new spirit worthy of their profession.

RESULTS OBTAINED AT THE *MATERNITÉ DU MÉTALLURGISTE* OVER A PERIOD OF THREE AND A HALF YEARS

Number of women prepared: 4,487.

	Number	Percentage
Excellent	893	18·43
Very Good . . .	1,097	22·63
Good	1,172	24·17
Total . .	3,162	65·23
Satisfactory . . .	859	17·73
Fair	595	12·28
Failure	231	4·76

The following criteria were used:

1. *Excellent.* Complete absence of sensation. Constant comfort of the woman who, throughout her labour, acts as during any everyday activity and adapts herself to her contractions without any effort.

2. *Very Good.* Criteria near enough to those above, but her adaptation requires a sustained effort and she does not feel as comfortable.

3. *Good.* On a background similar to the above, one notices at times a lowering of the threshold of pain, giving rise to a momentary and mildly painful character to the perception of uterine interoceptive sensation.

4. *Satisfactory.* Presence of an attenuated painful sensation occasionally hindering adaptation.

5. *Fair.* A state of psychomotive excitation which, however, presents a more favourable picture than the average one seen in the unprepared woman.

6. *Failure.* Restlessness and screams.

NOTES

ANREP—Professor Oleb Vasilievitch, 1891–1955.

One of the greatest physiologists of the first half of this century. As a student he came under the influence of Pavlov, who in 1912 sent him, during his university vacation, to visit Professor Starling at University College, London. In 1918 the Bolshevik régime drove him out of Russia and Starling helped him to settle in England. He became a lecturer at U.C.L., where he took a D.Sc., and became a Fellow of the College in 1928. He went to Cambridge the same year and was elected an F.R.S. In 1931 he became Professor of Physiology at Fuad I University, Cairo, where he stayed almost until his death.

BICHAT—Marie François Xavier, 1771–1802.

French physician who looked upon life as the sum of the " forces that restrict death ". He classified the tissues of the body into twenty-one different types (*Traité des Membranes*) and initiated the study of cell pathology, though he never used a microscope.

PAVLOV—Ivan Petrovich, 1894–1936.

Russian physiologist. He studied at St. Petersburg University and eventually became director of its Institute of Experimental Medicine. In 1904 he was awarded the Nobel Prize. He revolutionised the concepts held on digestion and the central nervous system. He defined the conditioned reflex and studied the laws that produced reinforcement and inhibition in such reflexes. As behaviour is determined by such reflexes, Pavlov's work laid a new foundation stone in psychology. In fact, in 1927, as the result of an accident at his laboratories in Leningrad, several of his dogs that escaped death developed neurotic symptoms, and this proved to be the first experimental observation of abnormal behaviour.

BIBLE—(Author's note).

Theologians have for many years defined precisely the meaning of the Biblical line: " In sorrow thou shalt bring forth children." The Bible, they say, is a book of history and there can be no question of anything more than an ancient observation.   In fact, there is nothing in the context of these words nor in the Bible that will lead one to give those words the tone of an order. The position of the Church with regard to childbirth without pain should be brought to the notice of all. Many of its dignitaries have shown their approval of a method which presents no risk to mother or child, the woman remaining fully conscious and taking part in the act. On 8th January, 1956, at a gathering of 700 gynaecologists at the Vatican, Pope Pius XII, in a long discourse delivered purposefully and with wise discernment, gave his full blessing to the Pavlovian psychoprophylactic method of childbirth without pain.

INDEX

ABDOMEN, 22, 93
Adaptation, 41, 45
Amniotic fluid, 88, 90
Ampulla, 84
Analgesia, 27, 29, 40
Anrep, 189
Anus, 83

BIBLE, 57, 190
Bichat, 104, 189
Bladder, 81
Brain, 33, 153–162
  activity of, 60
  reflex, and, 47
  uterus, and, 33, 62, 63
Breathing, 120–126

CENTRAL nervous system, 33, 41
Cervix, 23, 84
Cilia, 84, 86
Coccyx, 81
Contraction, 40, 41, 116, 127, 133–138
Counter-suggestion, 31
Cortex, of brain, 33
Cotyledons, 88
Cystic stage, 91

DELIVERY, 118, 138–141, 148–152
Diaphragm, 71, 124
Didactic method, 32
Dog, 48, 106

EDUCATION, 32
Electric current, 57
Electroencephalogram, 68
Embryo, 88
Embryonic stage, 91
Erofeeva, 33, 56
Excitation, 50
Excitatory factor, 48
Expiration, 124

FALLOPIAN tube, 83
Fear, 29, 65
Fertilisation, 87
Fimbria, 84
Foetal movements, 91
Foetal stage, 91
Foetus, 91
Fundus, 23

Goodrich, 30

HEMISPHERE, 51
Hormones, 84
Husband, role of, 99, 100
Hygiene, 93–100
Hypnosis, 21–23, 24, 31, 32

ILIAC bones, 80
Implantation, 87
Induction, 50
Inhibition, 50, 72
Inspiration, 124
Intercourse, 98
Interoception, 34, 52
Irritability, 46

LABOUR, 42, 132–141
  first stage, 142–147

MEATUS, urinary, 81
Membranes, 88, 91, 145
Menstruation, 86
Movements of foetus, 91, 127
Mucous plug, 91, 132
Multipara, 67

NERVOUS
  activity, 45–55
  system, 45, 46, 104
Nixon, 30

ONTOGENESIS, 33
Ovary, 83, 84
Ovulation, 84, 86
Ovum, 83, 87

191

ALONG THE OLD YORK ROAD

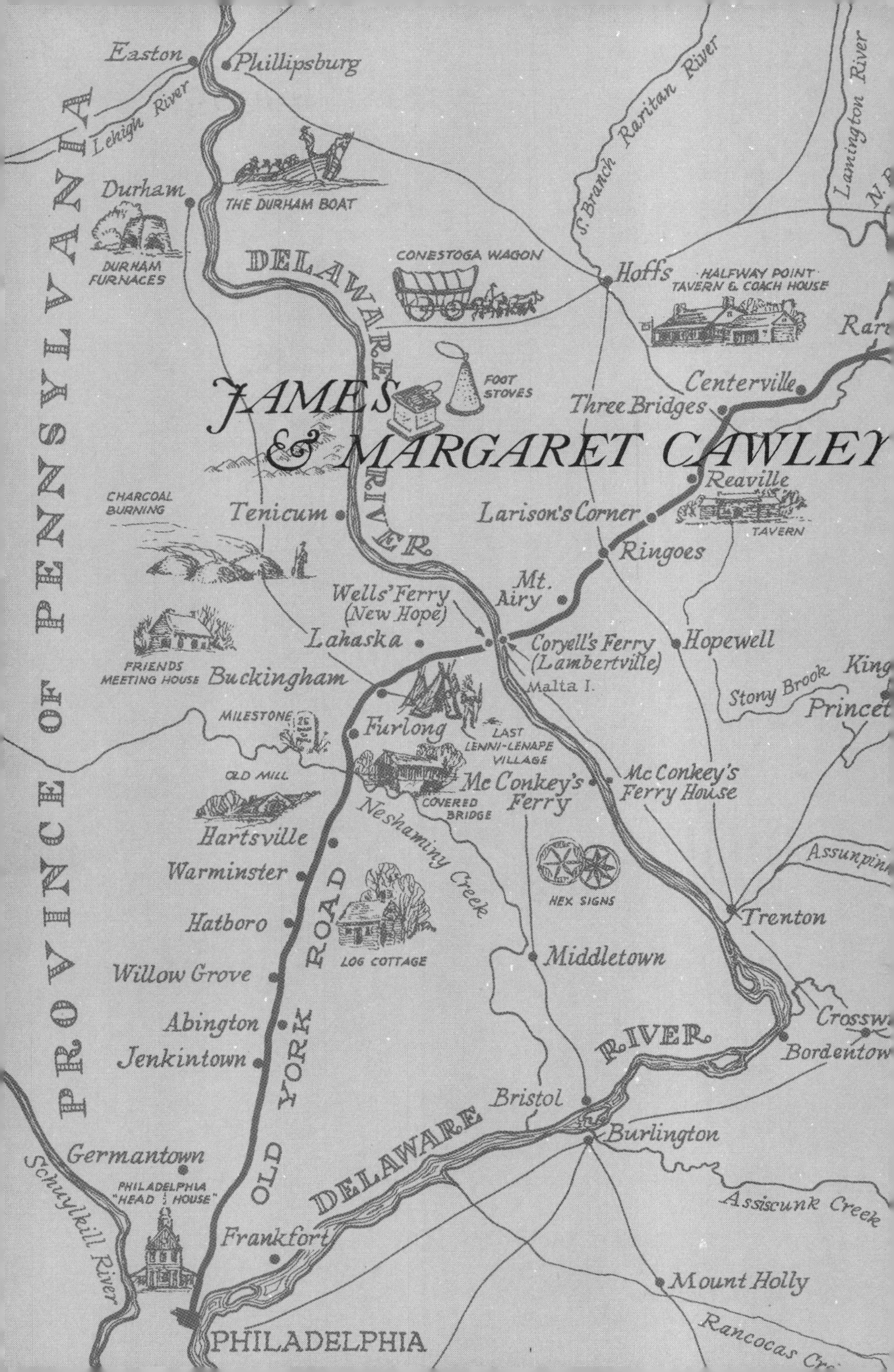
JAMES
& MARGARET CAWLEY
PROVINCE OF PENNSYLVANIA
Easton
Phillipsburg
Lehigh River
S. Branch Raritan River
Lamington River
THE DURHAM BOAT
Durham
DURHAM FURNACES
DELAWARE RIVER
CONESTOGA WAGON
Hoffs
HALFWAY POINT TAVERN & COACH HOUSE
FOOT STOVES
Centerville
Three Bridges
Reaville
TAVERN
CHARCOAL BURNING
Tenicum
Larison's Corner
Ringoes
Mt. Airy
Wells' Ferry (New Hope)
Lahaska
Coryell's Ferry (Lambertville)
Hopewell
FRIENDS MEETING HOUSE
Buckingham
Malta I.
Stony Brook
MILESTONE
Furlong
LAST LENNI-LENAPE VILLAGE
OLD MILL
Mc Conkey's Ferry
Mc Conkey's Ferry House
COVERED BRIDGE
Neshaminy Creek
Hartsville
Warminster
HEX SIGNS
Assunpink
Trenton
Hatboro
LOG COTTAGE
Middletown
Willow Grove
OLD YORK ROAD
Abington
Jenkintown
RIVER
Bordentown
Bristol
DELAWARE
Burlington
Germantown
PHILADELPHIA "HEAD HOUSE"
Schuylkill River
Assiscunk Creek
Frankfort
Mount Holly
Rancocas Creek
PHILADELPHIA

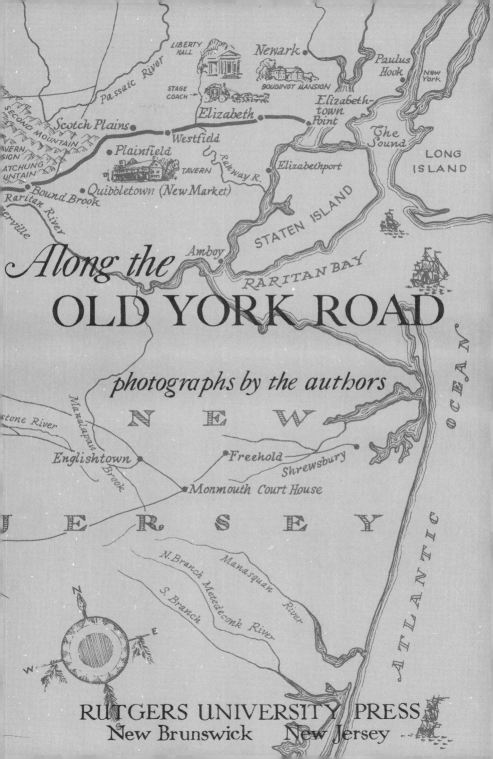

Along the
OLD YORK ROAD

photographs by the authors

RUTGERS UNIVERSITY PRESS
New Brunswick   New Jersey

The authors are grateful for permission to quote in this
volume passages from The Delaware, *by Harry Emerson*
Wildes, published by Holt, Rinehart and Winston, Inc.

For our ten grandchildren: Donald, James, Stephen, Edward, Jeff, Jennifer, Susan, Katherine, Jane, Kathleen, in the hope that they will always share our love and appreciation of their American Heritage.

PREFACE

The New Jersey portion of the Old York Road has always fascinated me. I remember it when, as a small boy, I was allowed to accompany my Dad on his inspection trips over the "long lines" of the telephone company that ran beside the road. We traveled by horse and buggy, and the journeys took all day. The quiet countryside, beautiful scenery, and the soft plodding of the horse's hooves in the thick dust of the road are still sharp in my mind.

I have a still greater personal identification with the old stage road, as my maternal ancestor, Peter Fisher, settled in 1729 on a 200-acre farm beside a trail that was later to become the Old York Road, near Ringoes. His original log cabin has long since disappeared, but the farmhouse he built twelve years later is standing. Carved in a stone of one of the fireplaces may still be seen his initials, P. F., and the date, 1741. I am a sixth generation descendent. The farm is now owned by my good friends, Mr. and Mrs. Kenneth Heston, who maintain it in perfect condition.

The York Road, or the Old York Road, as it came to be known in later years, was considered one of the most important of the few roads that existed in late Colonial and early Federal years, mainly because it was the shortest and fastest overland route between New York and Philadelphia. Thus our road not only played an important part in the development of commerce between the two cities; it also became the main travel artery across New Jersey, to which feeder roads were later built. The road was of great strategic value to the Continental Army during the Revolutionary War for the movement of men and supplies.

Our road is today a busy modern highway of blacktop and concrete and the high-crowned road of yesteryear is no more. But one may still savor its charm. On many parts of it there is the same beautiful countryside, and a surprising number of the buildings erected in Colonial days still stand.

The reader who will spend a day or so exploring the Old York Road by car, stopping for a time in some of the villages, particularly west of the Raritan, will find his journey richly rewarding.

JAMES S. CAWLEY, co-author

April, 1965

CONTENTS

I

The Early Years of the Old York Road

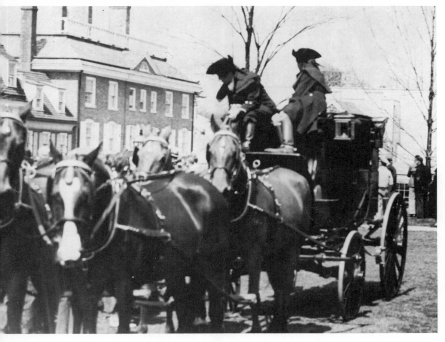

A replica of one of the more elaborate private coaches used on the stage roads of the Colonies. This picture was made at Palmer Square in Princeton during a celebration of the one-hundred-and-fiftieth anniversary of George Washington's journey from Mount Vernon to New York City for his inauguration as first President of the United States.

There is in history no agency so wondrous, no working in-strumentality so great, as transportation.—EMERSON HOUGH

The earliest highways in the American Colonies were Indian paths and the bays and rivers over which the Indians had been paddling canoes and dugouts for centuries. In 1664, the year in which New Jersey acquired its name and became a separate province, there were few roads of any length in this colony or in Pennsylvania, its neighbor across the Delaware. There was Lawrie's or the "Lower Road," from Burlington to the ferry at Amboy; another was the "Old Dutch Road," built originally over the Assanpink Trail from Elizabethtown through Woodbridge, Piscataway, and Inian's Ferry (New Brunswick) down to the Delaware where Trenton now is. A road also followed the north bank of the Raritan through Bound Brook, Raritan, and west to "The Forks," where the north and south branches of the river meet.

The first road of all, and probably the oldest commercial wheeled-vehicle road in the country, was the Old Mine Road, built by Dutch settlers in the early seventeenth century. The Old Mine Road ran from Esopus (now Kingston, N.Y.) on the Hudson River west to the Delaware River and south to the Water Gap, where copper mines at Pahaquarry had been worked by the Indians for unknown

3

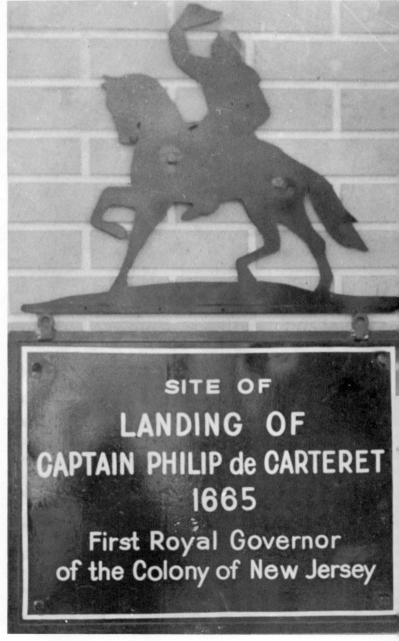

SITE OF
LANDING OF
CAPTAIN PHILIP de CARTERET
1665
First Royal Governor
of the Colony of New Jersey

Marker at the eastern terminus of the Old York Road. Here, at the foot of present-day Elizabeth Avenue, stage passengers boarded the ferry for the Battery in Manhattan.

years. Records of this road are scanty, but we do know that it was built by the Dutch because the Indians had no wheeled vehicles. Copper utensils thought to be made from ore from the Pahaquarry mines are in museums in Holland.

The York Road, the subject of this volume, had one characteristic that distinguished it from other colonial roads—it was built from west to east, to connect Philadelphia to New York.

The Pennsylvania section of the Old York Road had been cleared and roughly graded by about 1725, but for many years it was still too rough for vehicle travel. The whole of the road across New Jersey from Coryell's Ferry (Lambertville) to Elizabethtown Point was not open for vehicle traffic until 1764. Most of it did, however, exist in a series of local roads, trails, or paths from one settlement to another. The York Road in the Province of Pennsylvania appeared on a map published in Philadelphia by Nicholas Scull in 1759.

It is difficult, in these fast-moving times, to realize the physical conditions in the Colonies during the seventeenth century. Few of the colonists knew any region other than the coastal areas where the first settlements were founded.

As more immigrants came to the New World, the shore settlements seemed crowded to some of the more adventurous colonists, and they began to penetrate the interior lands. They had to travel over the Indian paths or make their way up the rivers. Some of them journeyed to the upper reaches of the Delaware and Schuylkill Rivers, using the birch-bark canoes and dugouts they had adopted from the Indians. Such streams afforded an easier method of travel than did the paths over which they could walk or ride a horse. It was not, however, until large grants of land were made to Wil-

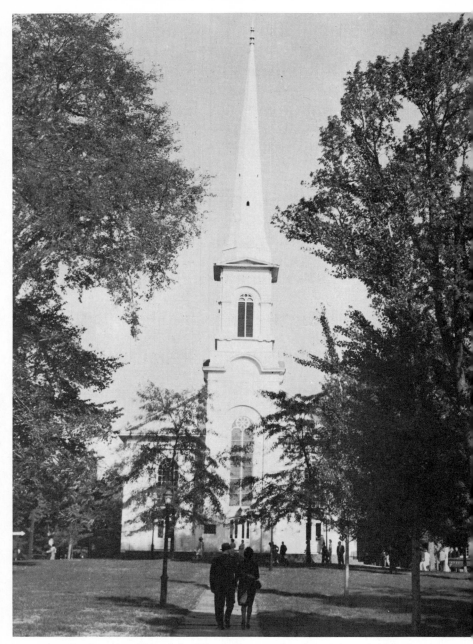

Presbyterian Church in Westfield, near the site of the original church
built in 1735.

liam Penn and Lords Carteret and Berkeley that any real effort was made to settle inland.

Penn's "Holy Experiment," following the acquisition of a substantial part of the Pennsylvania Colony in the "Walking Purchase," was the beginning of the settlement of that area. The land was heavily forested, and there were as yet no roads.

Historians are still debating what the actual arrangements with the Indians were for the "Walking Purchase." It would appear that the whole deal was something of a sharp real estate transaction, much like some of those consummated today. Thomas Penn, the son of William, made the deal with the Delaware chiefs who claimed they owned all the land along the Delaware River. The Six Nations Indian Federation argued that the Delawares had no more land to sell and that they could not therefore agree to the "Walking Purchase." To convince the Delawares that they (the Indians) were obligated to the Quaker colony, Thomas Penn showed the chiefs a "deed" which he (Thomas) claimed had been given in 1686 to his father, whom the Indians highly respected. In the so-called "deed" it had been agreed between the Indians and William Penn that Penn was to have "all the land a man can walk over in a day and a half." The authenticity of the document is doubtful, but Thomas finally convinced the Indians that they should honor it. Accordingly, arrangements were made to conduct the walkabout in the fall of 1737, shortly after the completion of the York Road from Philadelphia to Wells' Ferry.

There was a wide divergence of opinion between the Indians and the settlers as to what had been agreed upon in the "deed." The Indians interpreted it to mean a leisurely

7

walk, pausing for refreshments and ending the walk at sundown. In fact, what the Indians had in mind was a distance of about thirty-five miles along the Delaware River to a point where Easton is now located.

Thomas Penn had other ideas. He found three of the best young athletes in the Colony and told them to go into training and to familiarize themselves with the area to be walked over. They were told to blaze a trail so that no time would be lost when the actual "walk" began. An added inducement was the promise of five pounds in money and five hundred acres of land to the man who covered the greatest distance.

On the great day a group of Indians and white settlers met at the starting point. Penn's experts walked at a quick

Scotch Plains Tavern. The center section was built in 1737, and except for a few years when it was a private residence, has been continuously in use as a tavern.

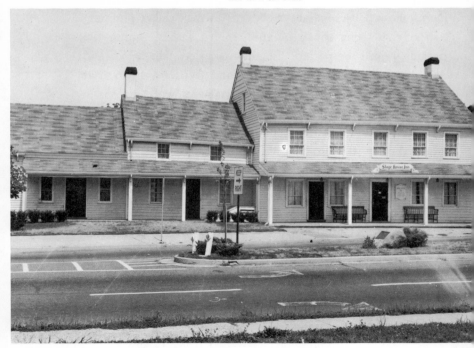

pace, actually a half lope, until the Indians were outdistanced. Then, it is said, horses were furnished to the white walkers, and riding a considerable distance on horseback, they left the Indians far behind. Even so, only one of the white men stayed in the race. He was Edward Marshall, and at the end of a day and a half Marshall had covered sixty-six miles, to a point near present-day Jim Thorpe, formerly the town of Mauch Chunk.

The Indians realized that they had been outsmarted but kept their agreement with Thomas Penn. In 1758, Penn gave the Six Nations the northern half of the purchase and the Colony paid the Delawares four hundred pounds for the southern portion. Thus, much of what is now Eastern Pennsylvania was bought by the Quaker Colony for about a shilling, or its equivalent, an acre.

Because of the difficulty of travel most of the settlers who bought land tracts in the interior had to journey to their new locations over the Indian paths, with only such goods as could be carried on their backs or on the horses, oxen, and cows, if they were lucky enough to have such animals. Strong backs, axes, and seeds for the first crops were the essentials.

As soon as the land was taken up the first task confronting the new settlers in the interior was the backbreaking job of clearing the land of the virgin timber, with which it was heavily forested except for some meadow areas along the rivers. The trees, usually stands of pine, hemlock, and hardwoods were difficult to cut with the simple tools the settlers used. As a rule the cut timber that was not used for the cabins, other farm buildings, and fences was piled and burned in the winter, when it was safe to do so. The burning of the timber made huge quantities of wood ashes, and this was the beginning of a new industry, the making of potash. The

9

settlers ran water through the ashes and evaporated the lye in iron pots. The resulting product was boiled with fats to make the crude soap of the day. Potash was in great demand, not only in the Colonies but in Europe, and all that could be transported to the coast could be sold.

Once the land had been cleared, the seeds for the first crop were sown around the tree stumps. Later the stumps were burned and pulled out, and eventually large areas of land were cleared for cultivation.

The first job after arriving at the land holding was of course the building of a shelter for the family. Trees were selected and cut for the building of a cabin. Other farm buildings such as open shelters and later closed storage barns had to wait a while. In many cases the first cabins were later incorporated into the more pretentious farmhouses as kitchen lean-tos. The building of a springhouse, at first of logs and later of stone if it was available, was an immediate requirement to keep meat, butter, and other perishables. Those stone springhouses may still be found on some of the older farms in New Jersey and in Pennsylvania. In fact, many are still being used, despite the general availability of modern refrigeration.

Before roads were constructed throughout the Provinces of New Jersey and Pennsylvania the larger rivers, particularly the Schuylkill and the Delaware, played an important part in getting goods to market. As the white settlers wanted to carry larger cargoes than could be handled in the canoes and dugouts of the Indians, larger boats were built. The most famous of these early cargo carriers were the Durham boats, developed to travel through the fast white water, particularly in the Delaware. The Delaware bateau, a shallow-draft, barge-type craft was also used to carry cargo.

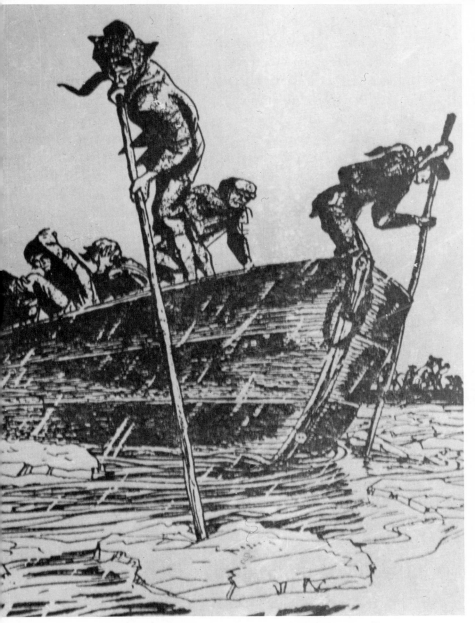

A Durham boat being poled through ice floes on the Delaware. (*Reproduced from a drawing, courtesy of the Standard Pressed Steel Co.*)

The very early settlers who took land in the open reaches of the Delaware valley were more fortunate than those who settled the interior in having a ready-to-use-highway—the rivers. It was the practice for years to store the farm crops in community storehouses such as Holcombe's at Mount Airy, New Jersey, until they could be carted to the river during the spring high water and floated down to the Philadelphia and other coastal markets. The Raritan River was also used in this manner by the early Dutch settlers to get their grain and other farm products to tidewater at Landing Bridge, above what is now New Brunswick. The Durham boats were not used on the shallower Raritan. Rough flat boats carried the cargo downstream with the current, and as there were no deep rapids, the craft could be poled back to the mills or farms.

The Holcombe storehouse at Mount Airy.

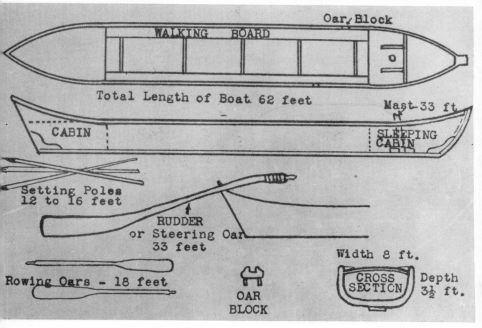

Working plans of the Durham boat. (*Reproduced from* History of Bucks County, Pennsylvania, *by W. W. Davis.*)

The Delaware in those early days was a deeper and rougher stream than it is now. Cutting the forest cover in its watershed and the use of water from the Delaware and its tributaries have reduced the volume of flow to a fraction of what it was two hundred years ago. It is probable that had not such a craft as the Durham boat been available to early settlers, the upper reaches of the Delaware and the Schuylkill would not have been settled until much later.

The Durham boat represented the first major advance in commercial transportation in the Colonies, paralleling but somewhat antedating the various kinds of cargo wagons that were developed as roads became usable for wheeled vehicles. Robert Durham began about 1750 to build these keel-boats, shaped like an Indian bark canoe, at his iron furnace near

13

Easton, Pennsylvania. They varied in size, the largest being sixty-six feet long, and carrying fifteen tons, and by the time of the Revolution there were so many of them along the river that they were the boats George Washington's men secretly collected for the famous crossing of the Delaware.

Successfully piloting such a boat, loaded with its cargo and crew, through the rapids called for expert handling. Of course the heavy cargoes were transported only during the time of high water. Even in those days the normal state of the water would not permit such commerce. The boats were of shallow draft and slightly rockered for quick maneuverability. A huge sweep was used at the stern for steering and along each side were hinged walkways for the crew to use while poling the boat. Those same walkways could be turned up and used as splashboards while running the rapids. A single mast was stepped forward for the sail when wind and water conditions permitted its use on the return journeys upriver. On the downstream trips local pilots were employed at some of the worst rapids. The fee for such a job was usually five dollars.

The return journeys did not require so much skill as plain brawn. At some of the rapids such as Wells' Falls, where there was and still is, a fourteen-foot drop in three-quarters of a mile, and at Fowl Rift near Belvidere, ring bolts were fastened on the rocks and the walls of the cliffs, to which ropes were attached to haul the boats upstream.

The Durham boats were used for a hundred years or more, and were gradually abandoned only after the building of canals in the nineteenth century. The last man known to have taken a cargo down the river in a Durham boat was William Lagar of Lumberville, Pennsylvania, in 1865.

14

So far as the authors could discover, not one original Durham boat remains today. There is a half-scale replica on display at St. John Terrell's Music Circus at Lambertville, built from the old plans by local boatwrights. Once a year, on Christmas Day, Mr. Terrell and a group of his friends, dressed in Continental Army uniforms, use this boat to re-enact George Washington's crossing of the Delaware.

The settlers on the rivers had easy access to the markets, using the rivers as their highways, but those in the interior were not so fortunate. They had used the Indian paths to get to their new land holdings and they continued to use them. These paths were well laid out and were easy to travel on foot or horseback but wheeled vehicles to take cargoes to market could not use them. The Indian paths, as the early settlers learned, were carefully planned to take advantage of the best routes to travel. The hills were ascended by the easiest grades; the solid ground instead of marshy areas was selected for the fords to avoid places that would be flooded during the spring freshets. It was such paths which were later widened to become early roads like the York Road.

As more land was cleared and planted, a need arose for mills to grind the grains and grist mills were built on streams with sufficient water flow to turn the wheels. To get the grain to the nearest mill the settlers hacked out rough "ways" from their farms to the mill. It was natural that as traffic increased other enterprises should be built around the mills—stores, taverns, a smithy, and other ventures to sell and trade with the farmers as they waited for their grain to be ground. Thus many of our present-day communities had their beginnings.

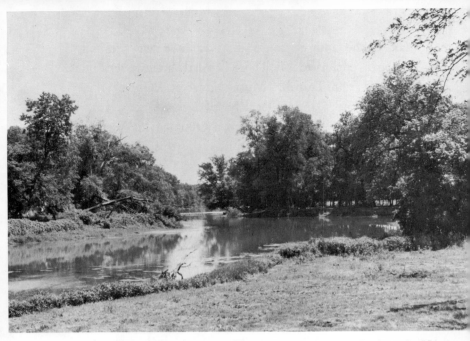

Tucca-Ramma-Hacking, "meeting place of the waters," where the North and South Branches of the Raritan come together.

Originally the farms produced only enough for family consumption, but as time went on, they began to have surpluses. A ready market existed in the coastal towns, if the farmers could get their wagonloads of produce to them.

As the settlers in both provinces felt the increasing need for land transportation, efforts were started to get their provincial officials to build roads. The Colonial governors responded by appointing commissioners to study and survey the best routes.

In the Jerseys, the first official step in this direction was the appointment, in 1675, of two men to "lay out common highways." In March, 1683, a commission was created to "lay out and appoint" in the several counties, "all necessary highways, bridges, passages, landings, and ferries, fit and apt for traveling, passages, and landing of goods." These boards continued for a number of years, thus laying the foundation for New Jersey's present highway system. No appropriation of money, however, went along with the appointment. The actual expense, which was mostly labor, was then, and for many years thereafter, considered a local responsibility.

In Pennsylvania, the petition of the Cheltenham Township settlers to the royal governor in 1693 was the first step in the building of roads in that province. This was followed in 1711 by the appointment of commissioners to survey the possibility of widening the Lenni-Lenape path from Philadelphia north to the Delaware at what is now Center Bridge. However, when it was determined that a shorter and better route would run directly from what is now Lahaska, on the original road, to Wells' Ferry on the Delaware, a new portion of the road was built and this later became the through stage route.

It was more than thirty years before the road was completed across the Provinces of the Jerseys to Elizabethtown Point. In the building of the Jersey portion of the road many stretches of existing roads and "ways," like the "King's Highway" and the River Road along the Raritan from "The Forks" were linked together. In a deed made at Ringoes dated August 25, 1726, reference is made to "the King's Highway that is called the York Road," which would indicate that the through road was completed at least to that point. However, it was not until 1764 that a survey of the road was made across Somerset County.

John Holcombe, who owned several thousand acres of land along the Delaware on the Jersey side, including what is now Lambertville, wanted the Jersey part of the road

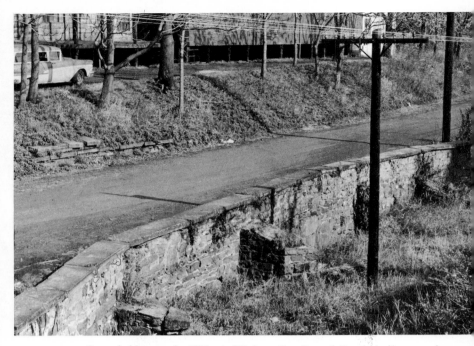

Stone bridge on the "King's Highway" at Bound Brook, built some time before 1700. The brook which it formerly spanned has been channeled aside. At the center of the bridge is the boundary between Somerset and Middlesex Counties, the eastern terminus of Somerset County's York Road Survey of 1764.

built over his land. John Reading, a man of equal wealth, owned a ferry a few miles up the river at what is now Stockton. He, too, wanted the road to cross at his ferry and continue over his land, and he had enough influence to cause the Pennsylvania Commissioners to lay out the road to his ferry at what is now Center Bridge. Holcombe finally won out and the Jersey part of the road eventually continued over his land.

While the "Upper Road" from Lahaska did not become part of the through route to New York, it did enable local settlers along its route to get to the Philadelphia and coastal markets. The main road from Philadelphia to Wells' Ferry then became known as the "Lower Road." A few years before this controversy, John Wells had obtained a seven-year lease from the Colonial Governors of Pennsylvania to operate his ferry. He paid an annual rental of forty shillings, which gave him exclusive rights to run a ferry within the distance of four miles along the river.

The Pennsylvania Road Commissioners were wise in their planning, envisioning as they did the future needs of the Province for more and better land transportation. In New Jersey, there was the same awareness of the problem, as William Franklin, the last Royal Governor of New Jersey said in his message to the legislature in 1768, "Even those roads which lie between the two chief trading cities in America, are seldom passable without danger or difficulty."

The Cornell mansion at Raritan. Section on the right was built as a tavern by George Middagh in 1734.

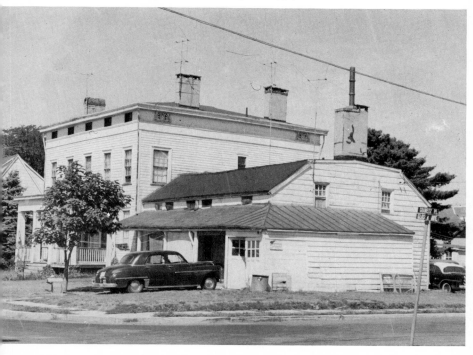

So, having recognized the importance of New York and Philadelphia as commercial centers and of more and better roads as the key to economic growth, road building and improvement was stepped up in the two neighboring colonies. In eastern Pennsylvania the roads, for the most part, were planned to connect the greatest number of interior settlements with Philadelphia and other larger centers. In the Jersey provinces the big markets were to the eastward: Elizabethtown, Newark, Amboy, and a few other communities.

With little if any road-building funds, labor had to be supplied by the farmers living along the routes. When the New Jersey townships were incorporated in 1798, local road officials were appointed and some funds became available. However, the farmers were still responsible not only for most of the labor in constructing roads, but in maintaining them. They were able in this way to work out all or part of their taxes.

The early road specifications called for a minimum width of forty feet, and there was some attempt to adhere to this rule. In practice, however, only a vehicle width in the center was properly graded. The farmers found that too much of their time was required, particularly during the planting and harvest seasons, to maintain their sections of the roads. To lessen their work many of them moved their fences in toward the center of the road, little by little, until only the graded center was left, leaving about half the original width.

In the spring those early roads, including the York Road, were all but impassable and a journey of any length was avoided unless it was absolutely necessary. This situation, together with the winter snows, left only a few months

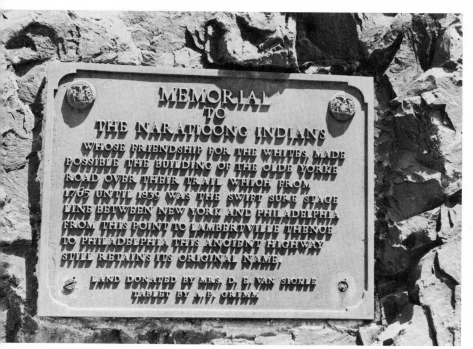

The Naraticong Trail marker on the Old York Road at Raritan.

during the year when the roads could be used by vehicles. Man on horseback fared much better.

When the York Road was completed across the Jersey provinces by way of Mount Airy, from the ferry, and on to Ringoes, Reaville, Three Bridges, Centerville, Raritan, part of which is now Somerville, Bound Brook, New Market, Plainfield, Scotch Plains, Westfield, Garwood, and Elizabethtown Point ferry, a vehicle road now existed over the shortest distance between Philadelphia and the Elizabethtown ferry. Vehicle traffic was possible over the portion of the road that crossed the Jerseys as soon as it was completed in 1764. Unlike the earlier portion of the road in Pennsylvania, the Jersey section utilized large stretches of roads already existing

21

and many of the old streets and roads between communities were incorporated into the through road.

During the latter part of the eighteenth century and much of the nineteenth, the increasing need for building and boat timber resulted in the spectacular rafting era on the Delaware River. Uncut timber was plentiful all over the provinces but the existing roads were not of a nature that would permit the cartage of the timber to Philadelphia and other centers where there were mills to cut the logs into finished lumber. A natural highway already existed—the river down which the timber could be floated in the form of large rafts.

The authors have over many years spent a lot of time canoe cruising the entire length of the Delaware and during those years have heard many and sometimes wondrous stories

Shohola, one of the rapids in the Delaware.

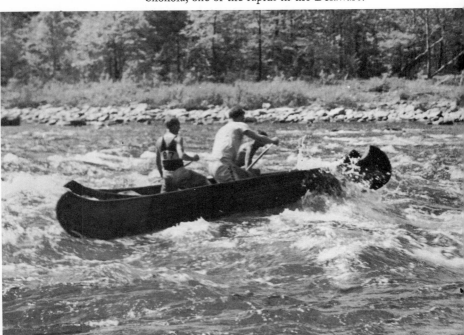

from old timers on the river. We were fortunate to have become acquainted with the upper river early enough to have talked to many men who had participated in the rafting runs and so much of our information is at first hand.

Like spectacular exploits everywhere, the stories got bigger over the years and perhaps also with the touches we ourselves have added to them it is sometimes difficult to separate legends from facts.

The great forests of the Catskills provided material for log rafts, some of which were over eighty feet long. To get such cumbersome affairs through the many rapids of the river required special hardiness and navigating skill.

The lumber used in the building of the Fisher farmhouse, mentioned in the preface to this volume, was rafted downriver to Coryell's Ferry and carted overland to the farm. Incidentally, the total cost of the materials for this large house came to about eight hundred dollars.

There are hundreds of stories, legends, and traditions about the rafting days. One of the more vivid descriptions is contained in Harry Emerson Wildes' book, *The Delaware,* one of the Rivers of America series:

"Britain's naval needs first led to a full use of the river. Shipbuilders on the lower Delaware, making brigs and sloops and small three-masted snows for the West Indian trade, offered markets for the loggers of the Catskills and for the husky raftsmen who floated the timber downstream to the Philadelphia yards. Lumber, therefore, was the first great industry to unify the people of the Delaware, and to bind all the settlers on the stream into a cooperative commonwealth. . . .

"The raftsmen were brawny rivermen, powerful with their huge sweeps, wise in their knowledge of the shifting channels.

Long before the Revolution had begun, shrewd Dan Skinner, admiral of the raft fleet, and Josiah Parks, his obstreperous bosun, were rafting eighty-foot pine logs from the Catskill foothills down to Philadelphia and walking back upstream through the untracked forests, with their pockets full of gold. . . .

"Each raft, before it entered the U-turn at Peas Island, tied up to receive its store of rum sufficient to make each raftsman drunk. Then, sending his happy men forward through the danger zone, where they would pole and push the logs, often while wading in cold water up to the waist and shoulders, Dan Skinner prepared a second rum supply to greet them after they emerged. Each raftsman knew that Peas Island was a place for heavy labor, but he knew also that Peas Island was the spot where he would get drunk twice. Instead of shirking the hard work, he looked forward to the crisis with gleeful anticipation. . . .

"Below Hancock, the raftsman's job was somewhat less exacting. . . . Dan Skinner's men were under orders to tie up for the night, liquorless, that they might start next morning, fresh and rested, for the passage of Long Eddy, for the swift run about Conchecton Hill, and for the passage through the Dreamer Islands, where rafts were almost sure to ground. Once past these danger spots, once south of "Lackawack," where the rapid Lackawaxen River flows into the Delaware, once over the dreaded Minisink ford, where whirlpools swung many a raft onto the rocks, carousing was allowed, to celebrate the safe voyage. The inns that lay below the Lackawack and Minisink were noisy with the songs and boasts and riotings of raftsmen."

All of the rapids mentioned in the account of the rafting days are familiar to the authors, who have run them many times in a canoe. This has been a favorite form of recreation for that peculiar breed of men and women known as cruising canoeists, and in our family it is of three generations' duration. Members of the Atlantic Division of the American Canoe Association, the Murray Hill Canoe Club, and others are still cruising the river during the spring season of higher water. Perhaps one could truthfully say that these generations have been of as hardy a breed as the raftsmen of old. Certainly the heavy white water looms much higher and more dangerous from a sixteen-foot canoe than it did from the deck of an eighty-foot raft.

As these passages are written, the authors are planning a Delaware cruise for the coming weekend. It is fall and the water will probably be cold, but the thrill of the cruise is just as great, in anticipation, as it was a half-century ago.

The Delaware River was the Elysium of the Indian tribes that inhabited its shores. Even today sites of their villages are being uncovered. The Trenton Museum doubtless has one of the finest collections of artifacts from excavations along the river that can be found anywhere. A chance find like the one near Kintnersville where a bulldozer turned over several skeletons is the manner in which many village sites are located. The authors had the privilege of working in one such "dig."

The white man, as did the Indians for centuries before him, came to love the Delaware valley, and, over the years, many legends, stories, and poems have been written about life along the river. One, "The Ode to The Delaware," by an unknown author, described the river in this manner in 1893:

> All powerful and restless,
> On it flows to meet the ocean

25

Flows the historic Delaware.
Not a jot its restless motion,
Shore, or rocks, or islets, spare.
As the untutored child of nature,
Down its rock-barred course wild
Forms it here an isle or rift:
Yet at times 'tis peaceful, mild
Still thou floweth on, resistless.
Flowing in, and out, and onward,
Ever gaining strength and force
As the fall, which rushing downward,
Swells thy torrent in its course.

Let us leave the rivers that were important when roads were few and far between, and go back to the third quarter of the eighteenth century. By then the provinces of both the Jerseys and of Pennsylvania finally had a through vehicle road from Philadelphia to Elizabethtown and Newark, with ferry connections at both ends. The first part of the road, from Philadelphia to Wells' Ferry, was not used to any extent by any kind of vehicles, except perhaps the heavy farm carts and wagons, until near the middle of the eighteenth century. The Pennsylvania part of the highway was newly constructed and, unlike the Jersey part, there were no existing thoroughfares to incorporate into the thirty miles of road. The removal of stumps and boulders left holes to be filled with dirt and they became mud holes during the rainy season. In fact, some of the places were so bad that split tree trunks had to be laid over the mud areas to prevent the vehicles from sinking to their hubs. At times the difficulty of travel made passage over the roads, except on foot or horseback, prohibitive until the mud dried.

All early roads were dusty in dry and muddy in wet seasons. By breaking the surface of the road at intervals with cross ditches on the steeper pitches, washouts were checked to a degree. Those ditches were known as "thank-you-ma'ams" and in addition to preventing erosion they served as brakes to hold the vehicles while the horses took a breather.

Today's motorist, traveling over these same roads in a comfortable car and driving from Philadelphia to New York in a matter of hours instead of days, finds it difficult to realize the discomfort and downright hardship of road travel in those days. Of course the passengers on the early stage wagons sometimes complained, or should we say usually complained, about the hardships of the road, but on the whole they accepted conditions as the lesser of two evils. They had two other choices—walking or riding on horseback. Actually, the so-called stages, during the early years of the stage lines, were not like the relatively comfortable and sometimes elaborate Concord coaches used after the Revolution. They were simply farm wagons with two or three crossboards for seats. For protection from the weather there was a canvas top fitted over bows. Those hard-riding vehicles could carry up to a dozen people, who had to sit on the crossbenches and usually hang on for dear life when the going got rough, which was most of the time.

As stage travel became more popular, some effort was made to provide more comfort for the passengers. Not much could be done in that direction as the wagons had no springs and the wagon body was affixed to the axles. With the invention of the elliptical spring about 1820 some of the stages were fitted with them. Still later, when metal springs were available, it was a bit more comfortable to ride in the stages.

As competition among stage lines became greater, such

luxuries as straw-filled cushions for the hard board seats were added. However, none of those early stage wagons could be described as being comfortable to any degree.

Most of the stage drivers were arrogant and couldn't care less about the comfort of their passengers. To hold to their schedules was the main consideration and whether the customers were jolted unmercifully apparently was no concern of the driver. Doubtless the increased competition for business later changed that attitude to some degree.

Reverting for a moment to the bottomless mud holes so frequently encountered during the spring rainy season on the York Road, there was a story told and retold by the stage drivers whenever they could find someone credulous enough to believe it: "While driving along I saw a man's hat in the middle of the road and I called out to know who was there. Answer from the mud, 'It's me! but take no thought about me; there's a man a-horse-back below me and he can't get out.'" With the established routine of a two-day journey by stage between New York and Philadelphia, the road became better graded and maintained. Traffic moved faster and it became the exception, rather than the rule, for vehicles to be delayed for road repairs.

From all accounts about the early days of the Old York Road it would appear that from the day it opened, particularly in the Jersey provinces, the road became a popular route for travel by an ever-increasing number of people. In fact, it is said that at one time as many as two hundred vehicles passed over the road in a single day. Considering the smaller population along the eastern seaboard at that time, the road would seem to have been as relatively popular as our present-day highways.

Frequent stops to change horses and the mid-day meals

28

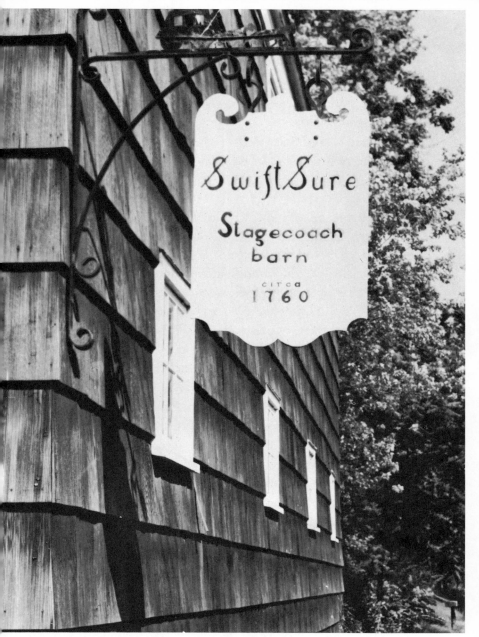

The original tavern barn at Centerville, now used as a community house.

gave passengers a chance to get out and walk the cramps out of their legs. Farmers made no complaints about the condition of the roads, as their growing number made possible weekly journeys to larger markets and a chance to shop and trade.

During the first third of the nineteenth century, private turnpike companies were chartered and many toll roads were constructed, in some cases near existing roads, but also in places where no road had been built by the townships. Through the sale of stock and the collection of tolls a good return resulted from many of those operations. Unlike today, the tolls were low and as a rule the toll collectors were families who lived at the tollgates. A long pole, similar to the old-time well sweeps, extended across the road and, when the toll was paid, the pole was raised to allow the vehicle, people, or cattle to pass through. Toll was charged for horseback riders and there was a head charge on cattle and sheep.

Many people still living remember the last of the tollgates. Some were still in operation as late as fifty years ago. Here and there some of the former tollhouses may still be seen along the highways.

As is sometimes the case today, people objected to paying tolls and there were all sorts of schemes thought up to avoid them. One of the most popular was the building of detours, or "shunpikes" as they were known, around the tollgates. Sometimes the farmer who permitted the use of his fields for this purpose would himself later charge tolls.

After the Revolution the more elaborate Concord coaches, that up to that time had only been seen in the larger cities, were put on the road as stagecoaches. Padded seats and strap suspension made them elegant compared to the crude stage wagons. Some of them were very colorful and had

30

the name of the stage line painted on each side. Many were in reality as large as tally-ho coaches, usually drawn by four and sometimes six horses, with a gaily uniformed driver on the box.

The years following the Revolutionary War showed a great increase in the number of stage lines operating. Their many vehicles, together with the long processions of Jersey wagons, Conestogas, and others could be seen going to and fro daily. On certain days of the week, it is said, some vehicle was always in sight throughout the length of the stage highway.

Freighting by wagons was an important method of exchange of products with other areas. Long lines of wagons carried great loads of farm produce. They were the equivalent of our modern diesel rigs. It is true, however, that much

Ringoes Tavern, built in 1840.

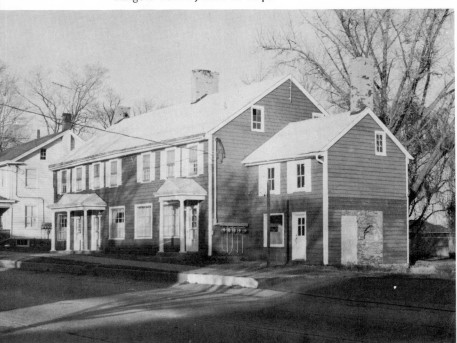

of the freight destined for coastal cities was still carried in sailing ships.

The outstanding stage coaches on the Old York Road were those of the Swift-Sure Stage Line. In 1769 advertisements appearing in the *New York Gazette or Weekly Post Boy* announced: "A new stage line is to be erected to go from New York to Philadelphia by way of Powles Hook from thence through Newark and Elizabethtown to Bound Brook and the North Branch of the Raritan to Coryell's Ferry, the only ferry between Newark and Philadelphia noted for its shortness and convenience over the river Delaware." Other announcements were that "Stages would leave the Barley Sheaf Tavern at eight in the morning, arriving at Wells' Ferry twelve hours later. There will be stops for refreshments and changing of horses every ten miles."

The ferry toll house at New Hope now houses the town's public library.

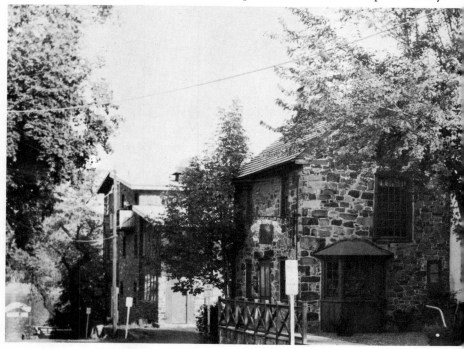

Still other bids for business may be seen in the following announcement: "Stages to leave the Bunch of Grapes at dawn on each Tuesday and the trip will take two days." By 1827 there were three runs each week. The fare was twenty shillings (about five dollars at that time).

Further emphasis on the desirability of travel on the Swift-Sure and other big stage lines could be found in the statement of the former that "Our route over the Old York Road is through the finest, most pleasant and best inhabited part of the state." Apparently, they were selling scenery as well as transportation even in those early days.

At first a trip was made each way once a week by the leading stage companies. Later on, when road conditions were better and more companies began to compete for business, three weekly trips were made. The faster and lighter coaches were more comfortable but they had one disadvantage. They frequently turned over and piled the passengers in a heap.

The Swift-Sure Line was a very profitable operation and it became more so when it was awarded the lucrative mail contracts. Swift-Sure held the contracts until the railroads took them over near the middle of the nineteenth century.

As is the case today with rail and bus lines, the fast through coaches were supplemented by the short-haul lines that operated as feeders to the main lines and for local transportation on the main lines. One of the short-haul lines operated between Flemington and Somerville in 1844 by way of Centerville and Readington. As a growing network of connecting highways developed, the necessary services in connection with the increased road traffic resulted in more villages along the highway.

The huge Conestoga wagon that was used extensively for

33

freighting on the Old York and other early highways was a very remarkable vehicle. Made in Pennsylvania, originally for carrying hay and other farm products, it later came into general use for overland freighting. Conestogas were designed to meet the primitive conditions under which they had to operate. There were few if any bridges, and road vehicles had to cross streams over fords, sometimes when in flood. The boat-shaped body of the Conestoga was built with flared ends and was so tight it would float in deep water and would keep the passengers and cargo reasonably dry when crossing streams. For really deep water, trees would sometimes be cut and the trunks lashed to the sides of the wagon to add flotation.

To keep out the weather a series of wooden hoops, secured to the sides of the vehicle, formed an arching frame,

A flatboat ferry and cable still in use on the Delaware a few miles north of New Hope.

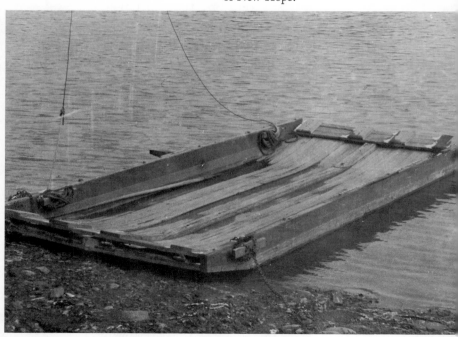

to which a white canvas top was fastened. Draw ropes were used to pull the front and back together. With the tops on, the rigs stood over twelve feet high. When ready for the road with their four or six horses some of those juggernauts were over sixty feet long.

The wheels of the larger Conestogas were six feet in diameter with wide rims for slogging through the mud. Under the rear axle were the tar bucket and water pail. Loads of up to six tons could be carried. This same type of "covered wagon" was the favorite vehicle used in the wagon-train journeys to California and Oregon during the early and middle part of the nineteenth century.

It must have been a thrilling sight to see the huge wagons and the faster express stages journeying over the Old York Road, up and down the hills of the beautiful countryside of Pennsylvania and through the farmlands of New Jersey. The scene was well described in a poem by David Ely:

> Many a fleet of them
> In one long, upward winding row,
> It was ever a noble sight
> As from the distant mountain height
> Or quiet valley far below,
> Their snow-white covers looked like sails.

There are many amusing descriptions of life as it was during the days of the stages. In *The Story of an Old Farm*, by Andrew D. Mellick, Jr., appears the following:

"Squeezing in on the front seat by the driver's side, our legs and feet were inextricably entangled in mail bags, bundles, whiffletrees and horses' tails. The stage is 'loaded up' three or four to each seat and, with a mountain of luggage

35

piled behind, we rattled down the main street of the town."

There were also plaintive little gems like the following, quoted from Snell's *History of Hunterdon and Somerset Counties:*

> Where is the coach? Where is the mail?
> The coachman, where is he?
> Where is the guard that used to blow
> His horn so cherrily?

Then there was the story of the roustabout who did whatever he could to earn food and drinks. He was known affectionately to the travelers who stopped at the Larison's Corner Tavern as "Gun." The cattlemen, particularly during those days, were a boisterous lot and sometimes not too thoughtful of others. It seemed that "Gun's" star performance to earn a bit of change was to get a running start, butt a wheel of cheese on the bar with his bullet-like head, and shatter it. One day some cattlemen, who had imbibed a bit too much, procured a grindstone and wrapped it in cheesecloth. This was placed on the bar and the unsuspecting roustabout rammed it with his head. After knocking the grindstone to the floor with his head he remarked, "That was the hardest cheese I ever did see."

Many such stories, poems, and legends became a part of the folklore that was built up during the early days of the operation of the Old York Road.

Another one comes from *The Story of American Roads,* by Val Hart:

> Oh, it's once I made money by driving a team
> But now all is hauled on the railroad by steam,

May the Devil catch the man that's invented the plan
For it's ruined us poor wagoners, and every other man.
Now all you jolly wagoners, who have got good wives,
Go home to your farms and spend your lives.
When your corn is all cribbed and your small grain is
    sowed,
You will have nothing to do but curse the railroad.

For those who may be interested in the folklore of the countryside through which the Old York Road passes, there is a charming little book called *Within a Jersey Circle* by George Quarrie, a visiting Englishman who obtained his material and stories, for the most part, from people living along the road. The book, which was published in 1910, has long been out of print but it may be found in some New Jersey libraries.

It is in this book that we find a vivid description of the actual sight and sound of the arrival of a stage coach. By present-day writing standards it is somewhat redundant but we would like to share it with our readers.

"One of the great personalities of the early stage roads, and in this instance, the Old York Road, was Colonel D. Sanderson. He was the owner and sometimes the driver as well of one of the biggest stage lines between Philadelphia and New York City. In the heyday of his coaching the Colonel's horses were the admiration of every one for their beauty and speed. He had the distinction of selling a pair of bays to the French Emperor for the handsome sum of forty-five hundred dollars. The transaction resulted in all probability through his pleasant and intimate relations with the Marquis de Lafayette who was a frequent traveler over the Old York Road.

"Colonel Sanderson's was a well known and genial face and his figure a commanding one as, seated on his raised 'box' with fares to the right of him, fares to the left of him and more on a second seat behind, he swung into view on the front of his glistening coach. Added to these passengers would generally be six or eight 'insides' and two or three more alongside the conductor, perched high on the 'boot' behind.

"Thus came the great chariot, tearing down the street of the town or village, behind the magnificent, foaming horses, spurred on by a blast of the bugle. The crash of the wheels of the towering equipage, the splendid connecting link between the two great cities of New York and Philadelphia, was inspiring and electrifying to everybody.

"To the passengers, whirled along by those nettled steeds, there was a sympathetic thrill of admiration and a sort of heroic fellowship with the noble animals, in their breasting of terrific steeps and their breakneck thundering down duplicate, rock-bound descents, with all the time, a delectable kaleidoscope of pleasant, pastoral scenes, forests, tumbling floods, sparkling rills and fairy dells. Then there was the exhilarating clatter of hoofs, the rattling, banging and swaying of the laboring vehicle, the merry whistle and the crack of the driver's whip, with his horsey quips and quiddities of stableisms, which the fuming chargers understood perfectly and responded to with the strength of fiery demigods and the docility of children."

No one of this generation is likely to experience anything like the thrill and excitement of waiting for and witnessing the arrival of a horse-drawn stagecoach at a wayside tavern. However, on a quiet summer day in such charming little villages as Reaville or Centerville, it is not hard to imagine

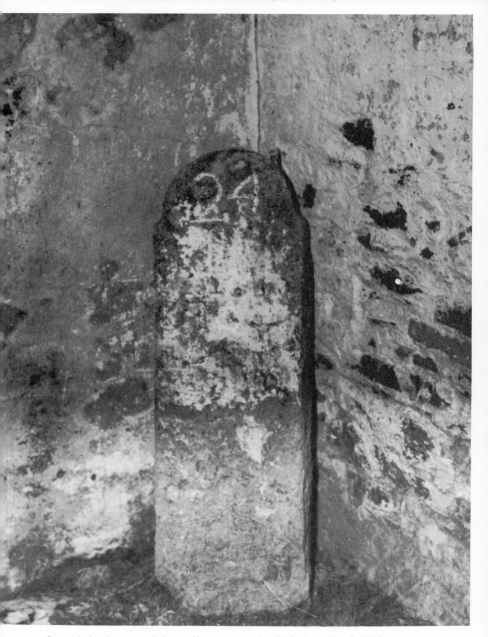

One of the few remaining milestones of the Old York Road. This one, marking twenty-four miles to Philadelphia, has been removed to a nearby farm for safekeeping.

that you can hear the sound of a distant bugle and the beat of the horses' hooves.

In 1764, when the road was completed across the Jerseys from Coryell's Ferry to Elizabethtown Point it resulted in a noticeable improvement of the social contacts between the residents of Pennsylvania and New Jersey. Both New York and Philadelphia showed a marked gain in population which in turn created a greater demand for products carried over the road.

Gentlemen of means sometimes preferred to travel on horseback and, in good weather that means of travel was doubtless more comfortable than bouncing around inside a stage wagon or the later stagecoaches. In the summer, however, it must have been a dusty journey, for not only the fast moving coaches but also light private vehicles stirred up clouds of dust as they whirled along.

Depending upon the condition of the road, the stages seldom arrived at their tavern destinations before sundown. Usually it was much later, particularly the stages on lines like the Swift-Sure that made the run between New York and Philadelphia in thirty hours with only one overnight stop. Whatever the time of arrival, the passengers knew there would be waiting a good hot meal, with a drink or two for those who wanted it. The taverns as a rule served good food even though the overnight accommodations left much to be desired.

Regardless of the time of arrival in the evening, all stages left at daybreak. In the winter, having slept in rooms without heat, the passengers seldom complained. In fact they were glad to get down by the fire in the common room and sit down to the huge breakfast that was the order of the day.

The great volume of travel over the road by private and

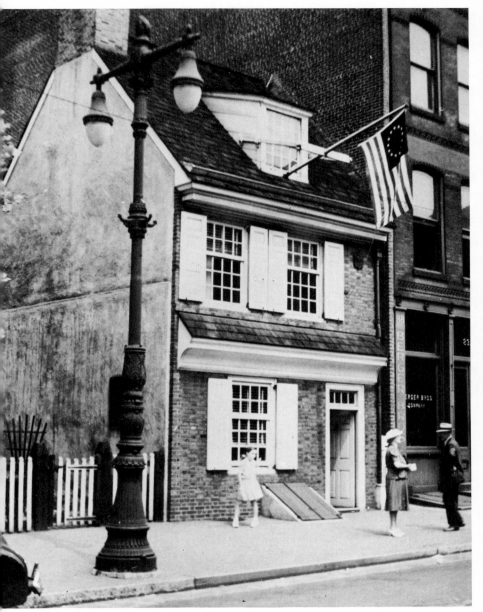

The Old York Road passed near the Betsy Ross House in Philadelphia.

stage wagons was a temptation to hold-up men, or road agents, as they were more commonly known. As a result, many men carried pistols to safeguard their valuables. However, the infrequent holdups of the public conveyances on the Old York Road were never as dramatic as those in later years on the western stage lines.

The principal revenue from the operation of the stage lines was of course from passenger traffic. When the mail contracts were secured, almost as soon as the larger lines like the Swift-Sure began operating, the lines were assured of good operating profit. It cost four pence to have a letter carried across the Jerseys.

The charge for carrying freight was a pennyweight for a hundred pounds and such cargo was usually carried in vehicles other than the passenger wagons which were lighter and faster.

During the heyday of stage travel the taverns, inns, or ordinaries as they were variously known, were vital to the operation of the stages and for the accommodation of the general public traveling over the stage roads. The overnight stop on the Swift-Sure line was made at Centerville for a time and later at Flemington, but with the best of luck the travelers on the stages had to endure twelve to fifteen hours of hard travel each day.

Tavern accommodations both for overnight and for meals varied a great deal but those generally to be found on the Old York Road were first class. It is to be assumed that after a day on the road the passengers were not too concerned about the accommodations. From Snell's *History of Hunterdon and Somerset Counties* we learned that, on the fifth of

March 1722, it was "ordered by the court that all publique houses in this county shall pay obedience and deuly observe And keep All the Directions of prices of liquors And other things contained in sd order which shall here After be exprest by the particulars, And that the clerks of the County shall record the same and give a copy to each publique house proprietor in the County. And they shall hang upe the same in some publique place in their severell houses, so that all Travelers And others may have Recourse thereto. And it so shall remain on the penalty of the forfiture of their licenses in case of default—viz., as follows, the prices all to be proclamation money."

Tunison's Tavern in Raritan (later Somerville) was an example of the better inns. With no modesty and, it would appear, somewhat disregarding the truth, this tavern adver-

Within the structure of the present-day Somerset Hotel, it is believed, is part of the original Tunison's Tavern, built in the eighteenth century.

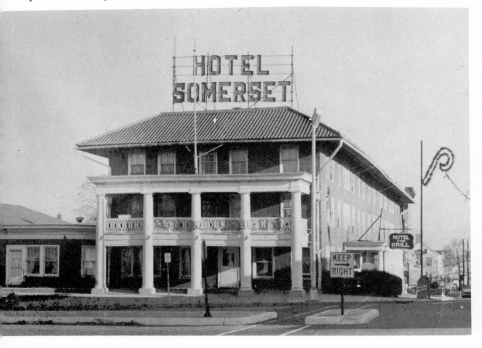

tised, "This is the only tavern between New York and the setting sun." Its published rates set by the court were:

> Lodging four pence; rum by the quartern four pence; brandy do [ditto] six pence; wine by the quart two shillings and eight pence; cider four pence; lunch one shilling two pence; horses stabled and fed one shilling, six pence; oats one half pence per quart.

On the site formerly occupied by Tunison's, at the corner of Main and Grove streets in Somerville, now stands the Somerset Hotel. It is believed that a part of the original tavern is incorporated in the present building. Today, as it was during the height of travel by stage, passengers arrive by coach at the Somerset Hotel but they have had a far more comfortable journey in a modern motor coach.

The typical tavern of the eighteenth century consisted of a large common room with a fireplace. It was here that the landlord had his desk and the room also served as a "tap room" with a recessed space and simple bar from which drinks were dispensed. There were also the diningroom and the kitchen on the first floor. There were several sleeping rooms, depending upon the size of the tavern, on the second floor. Some benches and chairs completed the simple furnishings of the common room. This room was where travelers and local people met in the evenings to gossip and exchange news of the road. In winter a fire was kept burning night and day in the fireplace.

The number of guestrooms varied. Usually several guests had to share a room and when the tavern was crowded, men and women sometimes had to share a room. Late arrivals had to sleep on the floor of the public room or bunk in the barn.

In winter the former accommodations were preferred as they shared the blazing fire all night.

The eighteenth-century tavern or inn was, as a rule, the focal point of the community. Town meetings and local business were usually conducted in the public rooms of the taverns. Legal notices of all kinds were posted on the bulletin boards as it was in such locations that the greatest number of people would be sure to see them.

Near every church a tavern could usually be found, and strange as it may seem in this day, the tavern, especially in the winter, was a necessary adjunct to the sometimes all-day services in the unheated churches. The congregation brought their foot warmers, filled with hot coals to provide some degree of comfort. Between the services the men would walk over to the tavern for a warming drink and be braced for another hour or two of worship.

One of the most popular and perhaps the largest tavern on the Old York Road was at Larison's or Pleasant Corners as it was variously known. It was said that "Sporting Corners" would have been a more appropriate name for this place, if all the stories about it may be believed. Frequent dances and other social affairs in the tavern attracted young people from as far away as Easton. In the winter they came on sleighing parties and on coaching parties in the summer. On those festive occasions the entire lower floor of the tavern would be converted into a ballroom by folding back the partitions, converting the several first-floor rooms into one area for dancing. The local tavern usually was the only building in the community large enough to accommodate such gatherings and, as the stage travelers were usually invited to participate, it made for a very gay evening after a day on the road. These events gave the tavern some social prestige.

45

A friend of ours told us that her mother used to drive in a buggy with her escort all the way from Flemington to Princeton, and dance until the small hours of the morning. The couple would then start the drive home, a distance of twenty-five miles, stopping for breakfast at Larison's Tavern near dawn. Today on our good roads such a drive would be a matter of forty minutes each way.

Larison's Tavern was rumored to have a somewhat sinister side. There was a small room on the second floor, without windows and with but a single small door. Poorly lighted by candles, it was a room of scary shadows. It was in that little room that the professional gamblers played cards with the cattle drovers and the more sportive local men. The "locals" and the drovers never won, of course, and never seemed to get any wiser. The room was heated in the winter by a Franklin stove and the nightly scene was described by one early writer: "The shadows cast by the candles on the tense faces of the card players created an aura of evil over the whole scene." It is said that large sums were won and lost in a single night's session and the games continued until dawn. The professionals would move on to another tavern to fleece a new crop of suckers the next night. When we stop to think about current investigations and probes into crime, times haven't changed very much.

Around most of the wayside inns and taverns there were acres of meadow for the herds of cattle or flocks of sheep the drovers were taking to market. Some of the cattle were driven to local markets from as far away as Ohio. In the summer a cloud of dust on a highway usually indicated a band of sheep being driven to market. This meant good business for the taverns and the drovers were welcomed, particularly in the bars, but the tavern owners very prudently posted signs in the rooms reading, "Cattle drovers must remove their boots before getting into bed." The cattle were bedded down in the tavern meadows, and sometimes were auctioned from the verandah of the tavern.

While many of the early stage taverns are still standing and, in fact, many of them are still serving the public as they have been doing for over a century or two, the famous Larison's is no more. It slowly disintegrated into a complete ruin and, as is so often the case with our historic places, it has been replaced with a gas station.

Edward Field in his book, *The Colonial Taverns,* writes of the intimate relations of the taverns, inns, and the old churches and the curious interdependency, one on the other, as local institutions. The roadside hostelries were known as taverns in New Jersey and New York. In Pennsylvania the designation of "inn" was more common. In the South it was usually an "ordinary."

Inns and taverns at times played an important part in the affairs of our country. Thomas Jefferson wrote the Declaration of Independence in the Indian Queen Tavern in Philadelphia, where he was staying at the time. Many stirring meetings of the Committees of Safety were held in local taverns and inns throughout the Colonies, before the Revolution started. The landlords as a rule were sympathetic to the American cause.

At Bound Brook, on the Old York Road, formerly stood the Middlebrook Hotel, first known as Harris' Tavern, when it was built about 1700. The tavern was known for years as one of the finest and most popular on the stage road. It was located near the Middlebrook which was and still is the western boundary of the town of Bound Brook and it was halfway between New Brunswick and Somerville. The early

Dutch settlers, driving up the Raritan Valley to seek land beyond "The Forks," favored the tavern, as did the travelers on the stage road.

When the railroad was built near the middle of the nineteenth century, it left the tavern in a corner across the tracks and a new turnpike added to its isolation. Ike Bennett, a veteran stage driver, refused to change his route and for many years continued to cross the tracks with his stage and dine at the tavern. One day his stage was hit by a train, and although he and his horses escaped injury, he drove no more. Ike never forgave the railroad for ruining the stage business and the accident ended the business of the stage line in that part of the Raritan Valley.

The Harris or Fisher Tavern was also noted for the fact that the first Masonic Lodge in Somerset County was reputedly organized there. During the Revolution it is known that Masonic meetings were held in this building from time to time. The tavern was said to have been the favorite rendezvous of the men and officers of both armies. Perhaps that is why it survived the war.

Some historians have questioned whether Harris' Tavern survived the raids and burning by the British during the Revolution. The building was still standing after the beginning of the twentieth century, and what was left of it was razed about 1917. Rings in the smoke-grimed ceiling from the British musket barrels could clearly be seen. The authors can assure the reader that this is a fact as we saw the marks many times.

Among the most colorful symbols of the early inns and taverns were the wooden pictorial signs that usually hung over the entrance of the buildings. During the early years of

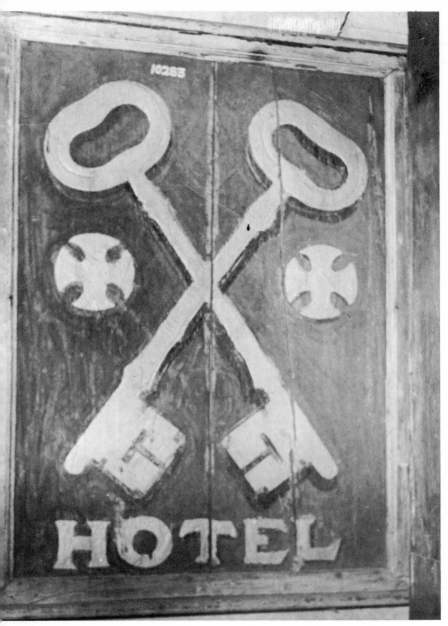

The sign of the Crossed Keys Hotel. (*Courtesy of the Mercer Museum, Doylestown.*)

the Colonies such signs were used by not only the taverns but other businesses as well. The pictures, painted on the signs— a boot, cleaver, fish, or similar symbols indicating the character of the business—served two purposes. One was for the benefit of those who could not read; the other was simply the desire for an attractive sign. For example, the sign might show a picture of a sheaf of wheat, and name, "The Wheat Sheaf Tavern." The "Gen'l Greene" sign had a portrait of that Revolutionary hero. Equally attractive signs hung in front of the Indian Queen, Logan's Inn, and many other taverns along the old roads. Some were truly works of primitive art. On occasion the innkeeper exhibited a sense of humor, as in the case of a tavern of somewhat unsavory character, whose sign had a beehive painted on it and underneath was lettered:

> Here in this hive we're all alive
> Good liquor makes us funny,
> If you are dry, stop in and try
> The flavor of our honey.

It is difficult to find those old wooden tavern or store signs today. Once in a while one does turn up in some antique shop but, like the one-time plentiful wooden Indians, it quickly disappears into a private collection or a museum. One of the largest and finest collections in the area is in the Mercer Museum in Doylestown, Pennsylvania. That museum, built in 1916 by Dr. Henry Chapman Mercer, contains what is believed to be the largest collection of implements, tools, artifacts, etc., with which the early Americans lived. These are well worth seeing for those interested in such things. When driving over the Old York Road from New Hope or Philadelphia it is only a few miles from Buckingham to

Doylestown and it is open every day in the week and on Sunday in the summer.

Though most stage travelers on the Old York Road preferred to end their land journey at the Elizabethtown Point Ferry, some continued on to Newark and over the Newark to Bergen road and the Paterson Plank Road to the Powles Hook (Jersey City) Ferry. From the ferry it was just a short trip across the Hudson to Manhattan.

On the journey across the meadows, passengers were frequently delayed because of the swampy conditions in places on the road. At times the stage would get bogged down to the axles. These conditions were improved some in places as on the Paterson Plank Road where split cedar logs were laid to form a corduroy road.

The vast area of the meadows, some thirty thousand acres in extent, was a natural barrier to travel between the Hudson and the Newark-Hackensack area for many years. In fact, on C. C. Vermule's official map, drawn in 1887, only one road was shown crossing the meadows. That was the Paterson Plank Road. On that same map Vermule indicates quite a number of cedar forest areas, one of which was the Secaucus Upland and Bog through which part of the stage road passed. It was from those forests that the cedar logs were cut to make the corduroy roads.

In 1764 a new road was built between Newark and Bergen, which connected with the Paterson Plank Road and thus continued to the ferry. Another and earlier road had extended from the ferry to Staten Island and by still another ferry to Elizabethtown Point. The Swift-Sure Stage Line used this route for a time until the shorter and faster Newark-Bergen road was built.

There has been considerable discussion among writers and historians as to whether the meadows are on the site of a prehistoric glacier lake; and whether, when the glacier receded, the land rose over the present area and left dry land which supported a wide variety of plant life, including many stands of white cedar. During our efforts to resolve this question we were not certain whether or not it was all a legend. However, through the help of a friend in the State Highway Department we were given a copy of a paper entitled "History of An Esturine Bog at Secaucus, N.J." From the careful research done by C. J. Heusser, its author, we are convinced that Lake Hackensack did in fact exist and that the land did rise and that it supported freshwater flora including cedar forests. In fact a dozen or so stark cedar tree trunks, blackened by fire, may be seen today from the Turnpike as it nears Route 46.

Many factors contributed to the final disappearance of the cedar trees and the meadows are now infiltrated with salt water, and nothing but salt grasses grow there. For many years, in fact, well into the present century, the salt hay was harvested and used for packing material in the shipping of fragile articles. It was also used to separate layers of natural ice when it was harvested and stored in the ice houses of the day.

With the successful application of the newly-invented steam engine to boats and later to rail locomotives, the end of profitable stage operation was in sight. The former sail ferries could no longer successfully compete with the new faster steam ferries.

The first steam ferry was named the *Raritan* and it was

owned by John and Robert Livingston, the backers of Robert Fulton in the development of the *Clermont*. Colonel Ogden, a member of one of the first families to settle in what is now Elizabeth, put his steam ferry *Atlanta* in service soon thereafter.

Considerable rivalry existed between the steamboat owners, and it is related that the competition was so keen that some of the captains of the ferries would stand on the dock and call to prospective passengers, "Right this way! Free passage to New York City, including a good dinner." It has a familiar ring. Remember the gasoline wars of our day? Soon the new steamboats were not only operating a ferry service between New York and Elizabeth; they also ran lines directly between New York and New Brunswick. Like all competitions, this new way of travel straightened itself out and those who had survived found it a very profitable business. The Vanderbilts and other business tycoons moved in on it and many fortunes were founded on the early steamboat business.

Some of the ferry lines, in an effort to take business away from the stages, made connections with the entrance of the Delaware and Raritan Canal, which opened in 1834, and thus travelers could continue in a leisurely way by canal packet to Bordentown on the Delaware. As a way of travel it was cleaner and more comfortable than the stages, but it was too slow to compete with the railroads that began operating soon after the opening of the canal.

With the opening of the railroad from Elizabethport to Plainfield in 1839, and on to Somerville in 1849, travelers began to transfer to the nearest rail point and thus the through stage traffic was lost, mile by mile. Railroads also

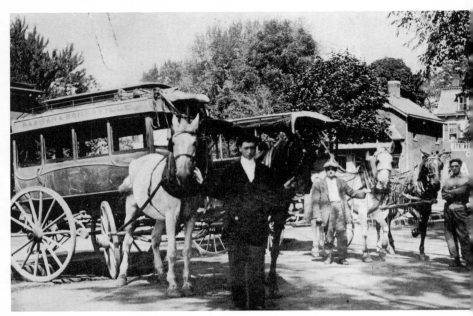

Stagecoaches of the Raritan & Somerville Line that ran until 1898. (*Courtesy of the Somerset* Messenger Gazette.)

took over the mail contracts, and this spelled the end of the colorful era of stage travel.

The short-haul lines continued for a few years, serving passengers for journeys between towns and from places where rail service was not yet available. One of the last of the stage lines on the Old York Road was that operated by Henry and John Frech between Somerville and Raritan until 1898. The extension of the electric trolley line from New Brunswick to Raritan ended the days of that stage line.

It seems so long ago that stages began operating on our famous road, and yet it is only a matter of a bit over two hundred years which isn't really long in the history of a country. The stage lines rendered a valuable service and helped to improve the economic conditions in the Colonies. Next came the canals and the railroads and then the electric trolley lines. Each brought better and faster transportation, each in turn eventually putting the earlier method out of business. Now the airlines are getting the passenger business with two-thousand-mile an hour supersonic jets just ahead. In some states passenger trains no longer run. Who knows what will come next?

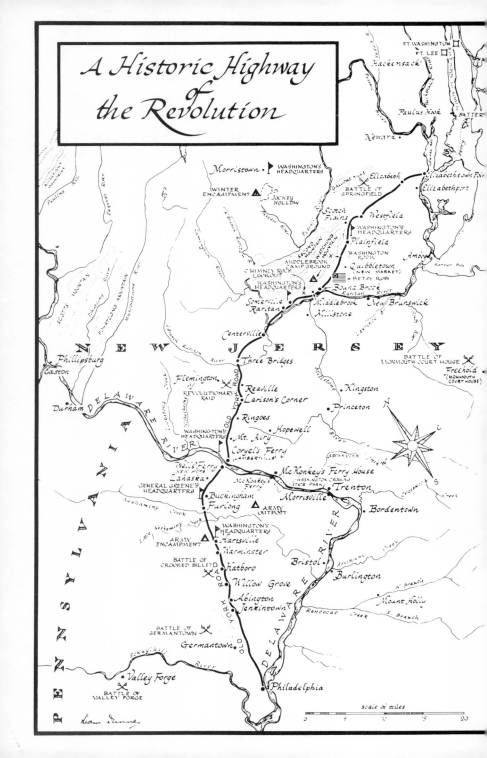

A Historic Highway
of
the Revolution

FT. WASHINGTON
FT. LEE

Hackensack

Paulus Hook

Newark

Morristown — WASHINGTON'S HEADQUARTERS

WINTER ENCAMPMENT

JOCKEY HOLLOW

Elizabeth

Elizabethtown Pike

Elizabethport

BATTLE OF SPRINGFIELD

Scotch Plains

Westfield

WASHINGTON'S HEADQUARTERS

Plainfield

WASHINGTON ROCK

Amboy

CHIMNEY ROCK LOOKOUT

MIDDLEBROOK CAMP GROUND

Quibbletown
(NEW MARKET)

BETSY ROSS

WASHINGTON'S HEADQUARTERS

Raritan Bay

Bound Brook

Somerville
Raritan

Middlebrook

New Brunswick

Millstone

Centerville

NEW JERSEY

Phillipsburg
Easton

Three Bridges

BATTLE OF MONMOUTH COURT HOUSE

Freehold
(MONMOUTH COURT HOUSE)

Flemington

REVOLUTIONARY RAID

Reaville

Larison's Corner

Kingston

Durham

DELAWARE

Ringoes

Princeton

Hopewell

Mt. Airy

WASHINGTON'S HEADQUARTERS

RIVER

Coryel's Ferry
(LAMBERTVILLE)

Wells' Ferry
(NEW HOPE)

Lahaska

GENERAL GREENE'S HEADQUARTERS

McKonkey's Ferry

McKonkey's Ferry House

WASH.-NGTON CROSSING STATE PARK

Trenton

Morrisville

Buckingham

Furlong

ARMY OUTPOST

Bordentown

WASHINGTON'S HEADQUARTERS

ARMY ENCAMPMENT

Hartsville

Warminster

Bristol

Burlington

BATTLE OF CROOKED BILLET

Hatboro

Mount Holly

Willow Grove

Abington

Jenkintown

Rancocas Creek

BATTLE OF GERMANTOWN

Germantown

OLD YORK ROAD

DELAWARE RIVER

Valley Forge

BATTLE OF VALLEY FORGE

PENNSYLVANIA

Philadelphia

scale of miles

0   5   10   15   20

II

The Old York Road in the Revolution

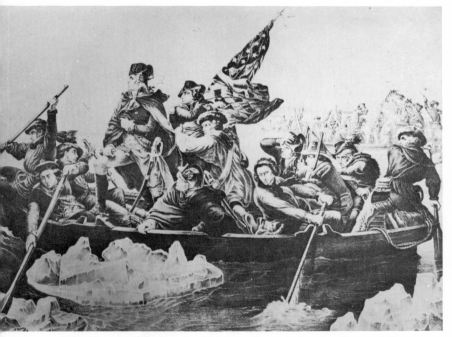

"Washington Crossing the Delaware," a painting by Emanuel Leutze, depicts the famous Christmas night crossing by Washington and twelve hundred men. The picture was purchased from the artist in 1897 by John S. Kennedy and presented to the Metropolitan Museum of Art, and is now on permanent loan to the Pennsylvania State Park at Washington's Crossing. (*Reproduced by permission of the Metropolitan Museum of Art.*)

AND HERE
IN THIS PLACE OF SACRIFICE
IN THIS VALE OF HUMILIATION
IN THIS VALLEY OF THE SHADOW
OF THAT DEATH OUT OF WHICH
THE LIFE OF AMERICA ROSE
REGENERATE AND FREE
LET US BELIEVE
WITH AN ABIDING FAITH
THAT TO THEM
UNION WILL SEEM AS DEAR
AND LIBERTY AS SWEET
AND PROGRESS AS GLORIOUS
AS THEY WERE TO OUR FATHERS
AND ARE TO YOU AND ME
AND THAT THE INSTITUTIONS
WHICH HAVE MADE US HAPPY
PRESERVED BY THE
VIRTUE OF OUR CHILDREN
SHALL BLESS
THE REMOTEST GENERATION
OF THE TIME TO COME

HENRY ARMITT BROWN

From the inscription on the Memorial Arch at Valley Forge.

The Old York Road from Philadelphia to Elizabethtown Point had been in full operation as a stage road for more than ten years when the War for Independence began in 1776. Just as civilian travelers had preferred this road as the fastest and most direct route between Philadelphia and New York, the Continental military forces early recognized its strategic and tactical value in the coming struggle.

In the years before the war, feeder roads with their short-haul stage lines and freight-carrying vehicles had increased the commercial traffic across the middle of New Jersey. During the first few months of the war, first the through stage lines ceased to operate, and one by one the short-haul lines also discontinued for the duration. Thereafter, until the war was over, the Old York Road was used almost entirely for the movement of troops and supplies, and by the couriers who kept the lines of communication open. This road, together with the natural fortress of the Watchung Hills, formed the basis on which Washington's plan to hold the Jerseys depended.

In the late summer of 1776, following the defeat of the American Army on Long Island, the Westchester reverses, and the abandonment of Fort Washington and Fort Lee, Washington withdrew his forces to the Hackensack Valley. When it was learned that the British were moving over the river with the apparent intention of engaging the Conti-

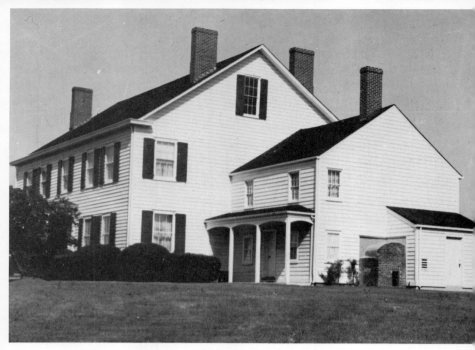

The Van Horn House at Bound Brook, now a clubhouse for employees of American Cyanamid Company.

nentals somewhere in North Jersey, Washington realized that his position between the Hackensack and Passaic Rivers might well prove to be a trap the British could easily spring. Following a council of war, it was decided that the American forces should be withdrawn from the valley. Washington directed the evacuation to and across the Acquackanonk Bridge and then on to Newark. Heavy rains made the movement of guns and supplies almost impossible. When the Continentals moved out of Newark and over the Old York Road to New Brunswick, the British were not far behind. However, Washington crossed the Raritan at New Brunswick far enough in advance of the British forces to destroy the bridge. For some reason not clear, the American Army stayed on the west shore of the Raritan and withstood a heavy artillery attack from the British. Later on, the retreat was resumed over the "Old Dutch Road" (now Route 27) toward Princeton. Leaving a rear guard of about twelve hundred men under General William Alexander, known as Lord Stirling, and General Adam Stephen, Washington and the balance of his force continued to Trenton. Having successfully reached the shore of the Delaware, where all the boats on the river had been assembled, Washington returned to Princeton to await events. The British soon crossed the Raritan in pursuit of the Continentals and continued their march toward Kingston and Princeton. Washington, Stirling, and Stephen, who together with twelve hundred men had been left at Princeton as a rear guard to protect the main army proceeding to Trenton, slowly withdrew to Trenton with the British in close pursuit. With his entire command on the Jersey shore of the Delaware River with all available boats awaiting the arrival of their Commander-in-Chief, the American forces crossed the river to the Pennsylvania side. It is said that the British arrived at Trenton as the last of the American Army was in midstream.

When the British learned that there was not a single boat left on the Jersey shore they withdrew to New Brunswick for the winter. They posted small forces at Mount Holly and Burlington, and a larger force of Hessians at Trenton. Many of the officers of the British army continued on to New York and more comfortable winter quarters.

Washington posted his forces along the Pennsylvania side of the Delaware River from Bristol to Wells' Ferry. The time was an unusually cold December and the troops had little or no shelter. To make it worse, many were ill. Few were adequately clothed and there was not enough food for

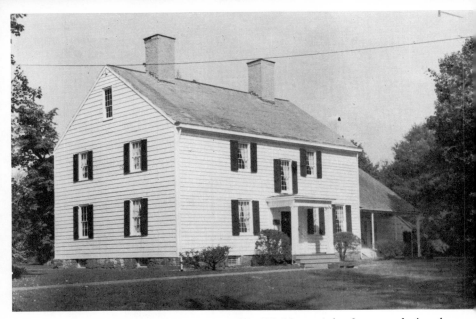

The Wallace House in Somerville, Washington's headquarters during the encampment at Middlebrook.

the men who had endured so much suffering—reverses in battle, long marches across the Jerseys, and an encampment in the bitter cold.

One bright note in the gloomy picture was the welcome addition to the army of two thousand Pennsylvania militia.

A stalemate now existed. The morale of the soldiers, and in fact of the people of the Colonies, was at its lowest ebb. The British were in possession of the Jerseys and General Washington knew that despite the condition of his army and the seeming impossibility of retaking New Jersey, he had to plan some dramatic stroke soon or admit defeat.

A council of war was called at the Thompson-Neely House, just a few miles below the Old York Road at Wells' Ferry. General Nathanael Greene, who had made Bogart's Inn his headquarters, rode north over the Old York Road to join the council. As soon as the officers were assembled, discussions were begun and they lasted for several days and nights.

In the meantime, Washington ordered Captain Daniel Bray to gather up remaining boats on the river as far north as Easton as a further protection against a surprise foray by the British patrols. The boats were hidden behind Malta Island, below Wells' Ferry. Thirty-five boats were secured and half of them were the forty-four- and sixty-six-foot Durham boats, in which horses and cannon could be safely transported.

Many plans were discussed at the council and finally General Washington suggested a stroke so bold that it seemed

The Staats House at South Bound Brook, later known as the La Tourette House. The center section was built prior to 1690. The house was headquarters for General Frederick von Steuben, Washington's inspector general, during the Middlebrook encampment.

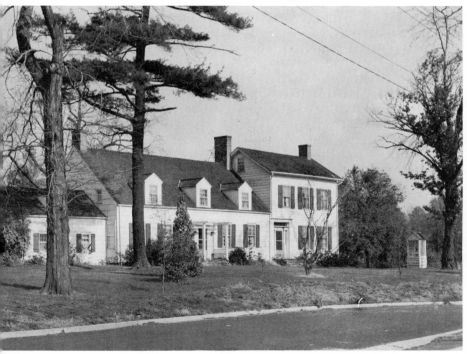

impossible of success. Washington's plan was to make a surprise attack on the British at Trenton, following a crossing of the ice-filled river at McKonkey's Ferry on Christmas night.

Preparations were begun immediately, and the crossing and subsequent victory at Trenton wrote a glorious chapter in American history.

To understand something of what Washington and his men endured during that bitter December in 1776 we suggest that the reader drive along the river road on some cold winter afternoon. Stand for a few moments at the actual point of embarkation and you will experience an emotional sense of history no mere reading about the event will give.

Every day, at half-hour intervals, a stirring narration about the "crossing" may be heard in the memorial building auditorium in Pennsylvania Washington Crossing Park. It will be an experience long remembered.

The magnificent painting, "Washington Crossing the Delaware," which hung for many years in the Metropolitan Museum of Art, is now permanently installed in the Memorial Auditorium in the Park. There are those who object to this painting, pointing out that it is not an authentic representation of the crossing; that the thirteen-star flag had not been designed at the time; that Washington's position in the prow of a rowboat is an impossible one; and that the ice-covered river is the Rhine, not the Delaware. All of this seems immaterial to the authors.

The picture is the most famous one of a series of paintings on American historical themes, done by a German-born American artist, Emanuel Leutze, in his studio at Dusseldorf around the middle of the nineteenth century. Leutze had spent an entire summer at Taylorsville absorbing the historic atmosphere of the area and he consulted with historians and official sources. This is not intended to be a photograph, but a dramatic conception of the most daring exploit of the Revolutionary War; it has become one of our national treasures, a cherished symbol of American heroism.

Near the Thompson-Neely House, a short way below the Old York Road at New Hope, which was Wells' Ferry during the Revolution, are the graves of many of the soldiers who died of disease or exposure during the encampment there.

Historians disagree as to whether the first battle at Trenton and the victory at Princeton soon after were the turning point in the war. It was certainly the turning point in the morale of the troops and of the patriots in the Colonies.

On the bank of the Delaware River in Pennsylvania's Washington Crossing Park lie the men of the Continental army who died in camp during December, 1776.

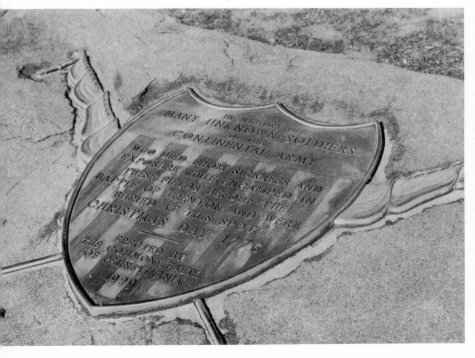

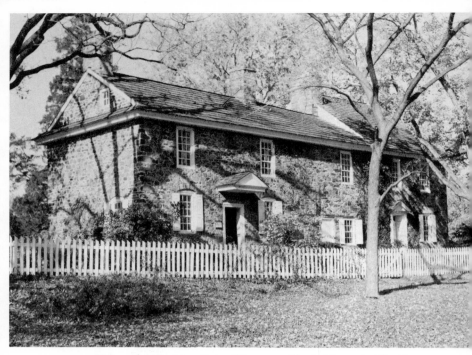

"House of Decision," the Thompson-Neely House in Washington Crossing State Park, Pennsylvania.

The man who should be the best judge in the matter is Lord Cornwallis himself. He expressed it this way at a victory dinner given by General Washington after the surrender at Yorktown: In a toast to General Washington Lord Cornwallis said, "Your Excellency, may I sincerely congratulate you on your splendid victory and may I say that I believe that when the illustrious part which your Excellency has borne in the long and arduous contest becomes a matter of history, fame will gather your brightest laurels from the banks of the Delaware rather than those of the Chesapeake."

Following the miserable winter at Morristown and Jockey Hollow, where the suffering of the soldiers was almost beyond human endurance, with snow at times over four feet in depth, Washington ordered the army to move down to the First Watchung Mountain. He had, during his winter planning, devised a new strategy, realizing as he did the impossibility of meeting the well-trained British in the open field. The loss of five thousand men at the battle of Long Island had proved this. Therefore, Washington decided to utilize the natural fortress of the Watchung Hills that extended across North Jersey. With few passes to be guarded and the Old York Road below, close by in the valley for the quick movement of troops and supplies to the east or west as the occasion demanded, the whole situation was ideal as a summer base camp from which forays against the British could be carried out. In addition, a nearby lookout, a rock formation extending out from the mountain, made possible a close watch of the British at New Brunswick and, in fact, on a clear day Howe's fleet in New York Harbor could be seen.

In May, 1777, the orders were issued to move out and the army moved down to the south face of the First Watchung Mountain, north of Bound Brook. Camp was established and earthworks were thrown up below to insure the army against surprise attack from directly below or from the east or west over the Old York Road. Back of the First Mountain near present-day Martinsville, two earth redoubts were constructed and a patrol left in each to guard against a flanking movement. With the passes well guarded, Washington had established an impregnable position.

In the meantime, the British were still in position at New Brunswick and beginning to send out patrols trying to induce Washington's army to come down out of their mountain stronghold and "fight like men." Washington did not accept

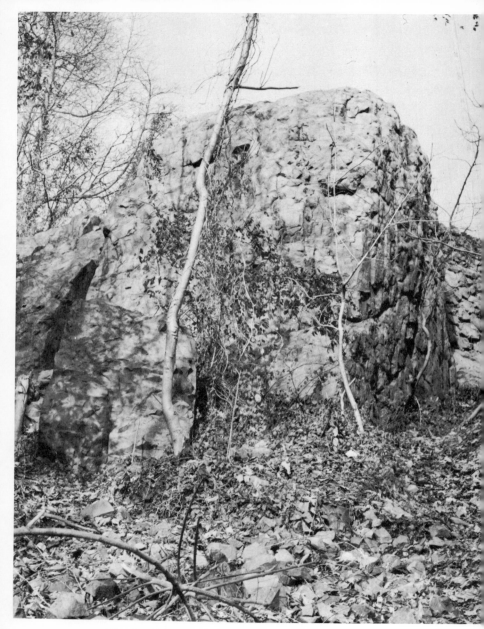

The Continental Army's Watchung lookout, now known as
Washington Rock.

the invitation and knew that he could continue to control the situation so that when an opportunity offered, his men could move to a favorable position to fight on his own terms. The value of the Old York Road in the situation cannot be over-emphasized, for fast movement of troops and supplies and as an easy route for the couriers who were constantly on the road.

At Camp Middlebrook there were only eight thousand men, of whom a thousand were unfit for service as a result of their suffering in camp the previous winter.

Having established his forces in the two strong positions at Camp Middlebrook and at the pass at Chimney Rock, Washington kept a lookout at what is now called Washington Rock to observe any movement of the British army or of the fleet in New York Harbor.

Apparently Washington lacked any positive information about the intentions of either the British army or of the fleet. At one point it appeared that the British were leaving New Jersey as they were seen moving to Perth Amboy and being ferried over to Staten Island. During the movement to Perth Amboy the British had to fight a rear-guard action against Morgan's Raiders, who harassed them during the whole march. By June 30, 1777, all enemy forces were out of New Jersey and it was again in possession of the Continentals.

Washington was still uncertain whether Howe was going to sail his fleet up the Hudson or south to Philadelphia. To be in a position to counter any move, Washington ordered his forces to move over the Old York Road toward Pompton Plains. If the British plan was to sail up the Hudson and cut New England from the southern colonies, Washington

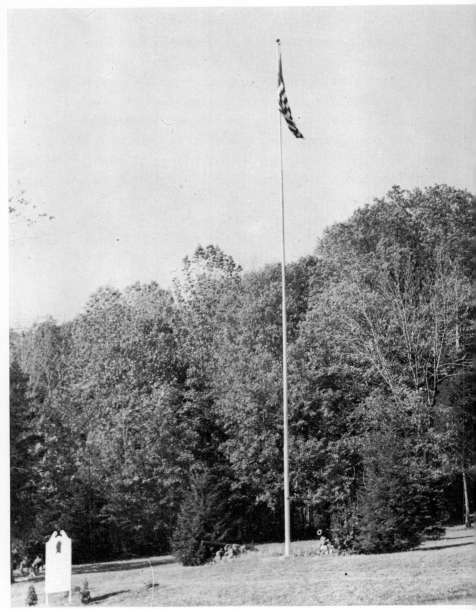

Camp Middlebrook at Bound Brook, where the thirteen-star flag flies twenty-four hours a day.

wanted to be near enough to the upper Hudson to prevent such a move.

The fleet was seen to move out, not up the Hudson, but toward the south. Washington ordered his troops back onto the Old York Road for a fast march across New Jersey to the Delaware River. He still was uncertain as to whether the British would sail up the Delaware to Trenton and attempt to take possession of the Delaware Valley or whether they would be content to take Philadelphia.

Having arrived at Coryell's Ferry, Washington sent Lord Stirling across the river to set up his battery and earthworks to resist the British if they made an overland attack from Philadelphia, over the Old York Road or up by way of the Pennsylvania shore.

Washington was quartered in the home of Richard Holcombe, General Greene at the home of George Coryell, and

The Holcombe House at Lambertville, Washington's headquarters in 1777. Lafayette was also a guest there.

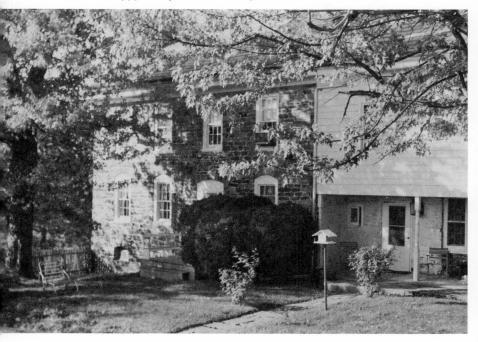

Generals Hamilton, Stephen, and Lincoln at other nearby homes.

The many errors of judgment on the part of the British commanders have been dealt with extensively by historians, but no one seems to have realized that by overlooking the value of taking possession of the Old York Road and preventing its use by the Continental Army, an opportunity to confine Washington to his mountain fortress was lost.

It has been argued that the British could not have taken possession of the Old York Road at any point because the militia and the patriots of the countryside would have prevented it. Possibly this is so, but we believe the British did not realize at any time during the struggle how essential the road was to Washington and that they therefore lost a good chance to pin down the Continental army. It is also likely that the road could have been taken without too much resistance because so many people of the area were ardent Tories and would have doubtless helped in the attempt to take the road. At least it's an interesting speculation on the possibilities, had it been taken and held by the British for the duration of the war.

While waiting at Coryell's Ferry, Washington wrote to Congress, then in session in Philadelphia: "Having received word regarding Howe's intention to take Philadelphia, the main body of the army will begin its march down the Old York Road toward that city."

Fearing capture, Congress fled to York, Pennsylvania. Thereupon, Washington moved his troops down to Germantown, five miles from Philadelphia, to be near enough to defend Philadelphia if Howe's fleet sailed up the Delaware.

Receiving no further information as to the whereabouts

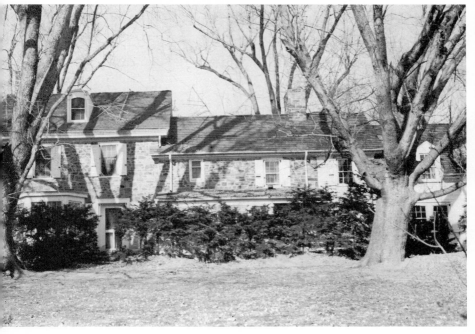

The Moland House at Hartsville, Washington's headquarters in August 1777.

of the British fleet, Washington withdrew his forces back up the Old York Road to the Neshaminy Hills, near the Cross Roads. He made his headquarters in the Moland House and the army camped along the road.

The Continental army at this point were not the raw, untrained troops of a year earlier. The majority were seasoned veterans. Even the militia units were trained and hardened in combat and could give a good account of themselves in battle, as it became apparent at the battle of the Brandywine and at Germantown.

For nearly two weeks Washington stayed at his headquarters at the Cross Roads, waiting for information as to the whereabouts of the British fleet. Word was finally received that the fleet had been sighted off the Maryland coast in Chesapeake Bay. He then issued the following order:

GENERAL ORDERS

The Cross Roads Headquarters
August 21, 1777

The whole army is to march tomorrow morning, the General to beat at half past three; the Troop at half past four and at five o'clock the troops begin their march. The Major Generals, Quarter Master General and the Commissary General will receive their orders at Headquarters at five o'clock this afternoon. An orderly man from each regiment of horse to attend at that time for orders.

George Washington
Commander-in-Chief

With the army on the march down the Old York Road to Philadelphia was the young Frenchman, the Marquis de Lafayette, who had been sworn in as a major general at the Moland House headquarters the day before by General Washington.

Washington had two objectives in mind for the march to Philadelphia. One was to quiet the fears of the populace, who had heard that the British were on their way to take the city. Washington believed that by parading his entire army through the city he could stiffen the morale of the people. His other thought was to plan to meet the British outside the city and to defend it against invasion. When it was learned that Howe apparently was going to land his troops at the head of Chesapeake Bay, instead of at some point such as Chester on the Delaware, Washington decided to precipitate the battle at a point of his own choice. The place he

74

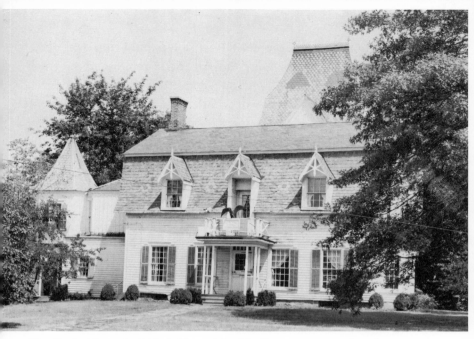

The Drake House in Plainfield, used by Washington as a meeting place with his spies and scouts, has been restored by local organizations and is now a museum.

selected was Chadd's Ford on Brandywine Creek. The result of that encounter could be considered a draw as Washington, despite his immediate loss, was able to withdraw to the safety of the Schuylkill hills.

At the beginning of October, Washington decided to try again to draw the British out of Philadelphia, which they had occupied following their victory at Brandywine. Four lines of troops were moved down the Bethlehem Pike and the Old York Road toward Germantown. Washington hoped to encircle the British when they came out of Philadelphia to meet him.

Germantown turned out to be another Brandywine, for on October 4, 1777, the tide of battle turned against the

75

Continentals and, despite the valiant account they had given of their ability to fight, the American forces had to break off the engagement and move out. Again the Old York Road enabled the army to withdraw successfully some of the command east over the roads about twenty miles before they made camp near Pennypacker's Mill. The nearness of the Old York Road to Valley Forge was an important factor when the army went into camp that winter.

While the army was suffering from lack of food and clothing and stricken with disease during that terrible winter at Valley Forge another condition added to their misery. It was the great number of Tories along the Old York Road, particularly those who sold their farm products to the British in Philadelphia instead of to the starving Americans. There were not enough men in good health to man patrols to stop the practice.

In the middle of the winter, or so it seemed, Washington wrote the following letter to Congress. It was dated December 23, 1777.

> I am now convinced without a doubt, that unless some great change suddenly takes place . . . this army must inevitably be reduced to one or other of these three things. Starve, dissolve or disperse, in order to obtain subsistence in the best manner they can: rest assured Sirs this is not an exaggerated picture, but that I have abundant reason to support what I say.

British foraging parties constantly raided farms along the Old York Road and those patriots who held out farm products for the American forces were treated harshly by the raiding British. Less and less food was available for the starving troops at Valley Forge.

76

Cattle were driven over the Old York Road from other areas and, when they could get them through to the camp at Valley Forge, the troops could have meat. One cattle drover, with a good-sized herd of cattle, asked General Lacey for a military escort as he neared Hatboro. The drover feared the British raiding parties would capture the desperately needed cattle. Lacey refused because he could not spare any of his command for escort duty. As a result, when the drover with his precious cattle had left the Old York Road and were only a few miles from the camp, the cattle were confiscated by a British raiding party.

Both British and the American patrols constantly searched the countryside for supplies, but food of all kinds was scarce. Lacey did his best with his small command to stop the smuggling of food into Philadelphia. All roads leading into Philadelphia were patrolled, particularly the Old York Road over which most of the supplies were going. On several occasions Lacey and his small force barely escaped capture, when they operated too close to the British lines.

Thomas Paine well reflected the feeling of the desperate men at Valley Forge when he wrote: "These are the times that try men's souls; the summer soldier and the sunshine patriot will, in this crisis, shrink from the service of their country; but he that stands it now deserves the love and thanks of men and women. Tyranny, like hell, is not easily conquered.

"Yet we have this consolation with us, that the harder the conflict, the more glorious the triumph."

Some historians contend that the suffering at Valley Forge, during the winter of 1777-78, was due largely to the inefficient management of the Commissary General Joseph Trumbull of Connecticut. A more important factor was that

77

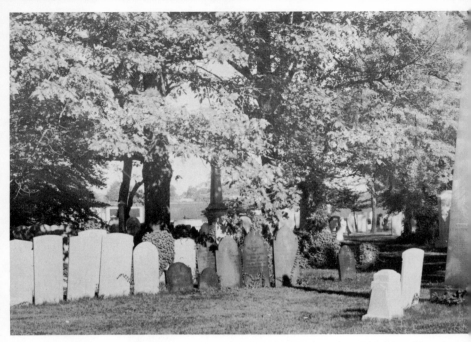

Graves of Revolutionary soldiers in the churchyard of Old First Church in Elizabeth.

both the British in Philadelphia and the American forces at Valley Forge were trying to live that winter off of a small area of countryside that had been stripped almost bare of food.

General Lacey and his patrol were trying to seal off Hatboro, where the Tories were still successfully getting food to the British, and one night the General and his four hundred men were in camp near the Crooked Billet Tavern. Early in the morning of May 1, 1778, a large British patrol that had been tipped off as to Lacey's whereabouts surprised the American force, and before that skirmish, as it is known in history, was over, it had cost Lacey twenty-six men killed and twenty-eight wounded and missing. Fighting a rear-guard action,

Lacey was able to save his command and they retired up the Old York Road. As a result the British held the Old York Road as far east as the Cross Roads, near the Neshaminy.

When word of the disastrous engagement reached Washington at Valley Forge he again wrote to Congress at York. "Every kind of villainy is carried on by the people near the enemy lines and, from their general conduct, I am induced to believe that but few real friends to America are left within ten miles of Philadelphia."

With the coming of spring, conditions were somewhat better at the Valley Forge encampment. Lacey had gained possession again of the Old York Road to a point below Hatboro and, in response to Washington's desperate pleas, cattle were moved in from western Pennsylvania and the Jersey

Replicas of the log huts in which Continental soldiers lived during the winter at Valley Forge.

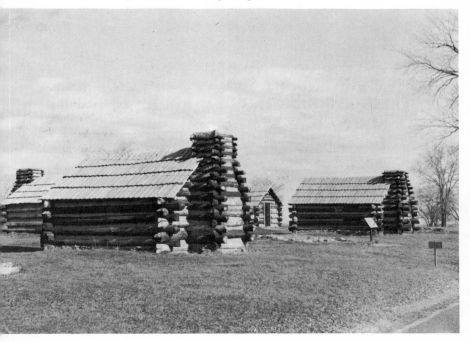

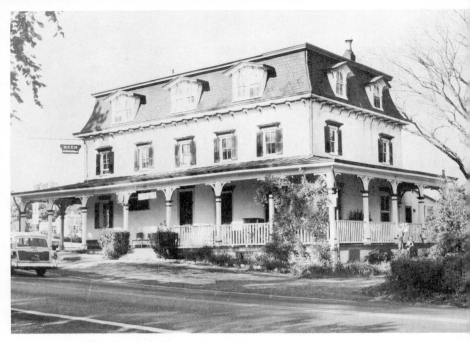

The General Greene Inn at Buckingham Crossing, originally Bogart's Tavern. The first Bucks County Committee for Safety met here, and it was General Greene's headquarters in 1776.

provinces. For the first time there was enough food for the troops.

When word was received in the spring of 1778 of the intention of the British to evacuate Philadelphia, Washington decided to follow on a route over the Old York Road to Wells' Ferry that would put his forces close enough to engage the British. The British moved out in mid-June, over the road to Bristol and across the Delaware River at that point, with the apparent intention of crossing the Jerseys.

On June 19th, Washington ordered General Charles Lee and his six brigades to march to Wells' Ferry. Lafayette and Baron de Kalb were to follow the next day with Washington and the balance of the troops. All the forces of weather hampered that march. Rain had so mired the Old York Road that it was almost impossible to move the guns over it. The General was forced to stop overnight at Buckingham. He arrived at Coryell's Ferry on June 21st. Lee and his men had crossed the Delaware at that point the night before and were proceeding toward Hopewell in Jersey, having dragged their guns by main strength up over Goat Hill Road from Coryell's Ferry. Even today, with the modern road that surmounts that hill, the grades are terrific. One can well visualize what an almost superhuman task it must have been to get horses and guns over the road as it was during that stormy night in June, 1778.

Daniel Morgan and his raiders were ordered down the Delaware Valley to locate the British and harass their rear.

The events of the meeting of the two armies near Mon-

Friends' Meetinghouse at Lahaska, built in 1768, and used as a military hospital during the Revolution.

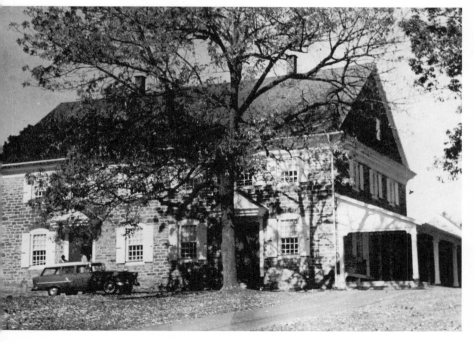

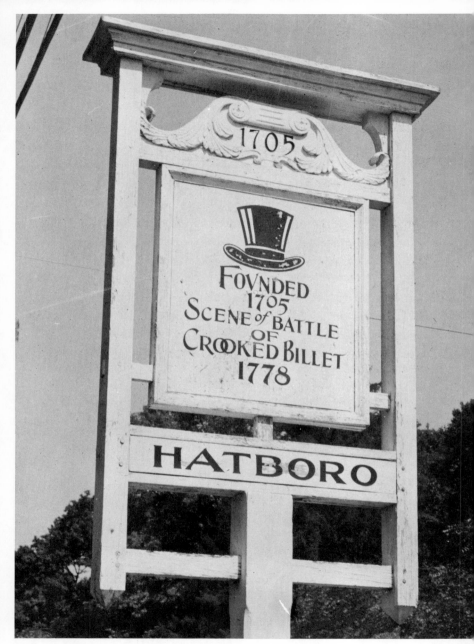

1705

FOVNDED
1705
SCENE of BATTLE
OF
CROOKED BILLET
1778

HATBORO

General John Lacey and his patrol of four hundred men were ambushed
here and severely mauled in a night-time battle.

mouth Court House are too well known to repeat here. However, it was once again the Old York Road that made possible the quick march of the Army from Valley Forge to the battlefield. While the battle was not a clear-cut victory for the Continentals, it did again boost the morale of the troops.

As the final days of the epic struggle for independence made the American people more confident of eventual success, the now hardened and confident army moved south to Virginia. The surrender of the British at Yorktown was the final act in the long struggle for freedom for which the men of the Continental army and the militia of the various Colonies had fought so long and so hard.

On a tablet in the memorial tower at Bowman's Hill in Washington Crossing Park is inscribed a short tribute that aptly sums up the feeling of the American people following the victory and surrender at Yorktown:

It may be doubted whether so small a number of men ever employed so short a space of time with greater or more lasting results upon the history of the world.

Does it sound familiar? We wonder if it could have possibly inspired the famous statement of Winston Churchill during World War II when he said, "Never in the field of human conflict was so much owed by so many to so few."

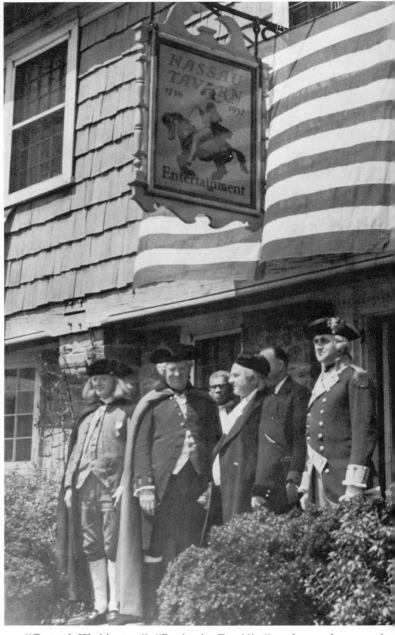

"General Washington," "Benjamin Franklin," and attendants at the Nassau Tavern in Princeton during the re-enactment in 1939 of Washington's coach journey to New York for his inauguration.

III

The Old York Road Today

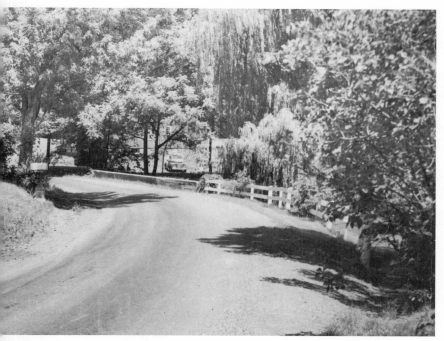

The Old York Road at Centerville. Here in this pre-Revolutionary village are many reminders of the days when the local tavern was the overnight stop for the Swift-Sure stagecoaches.

The authors, having enjoyed so many interesting days exploring the Old York Road, hope that their readers will also want to see the many historic places on this highway of the past. For those who enjoy, as we do, spending a summer day wandering along an old road, stopping here and there to savor the charm of things and places of an earlier day, a personally guided tour over the Old York Road would be in order. So come along and let us tell you about it. On an exploring trip like this, one should not hurry. Perhaps several days should be devoted to it.

Our highway can be explored with the starting point at either end, whichever is most convenient. Doubtless the people of New Jersey will want to start their exploration at Elizabeth and continue over the entire road to Front and Arch Streets in Philadelphia. Others may prefer to reverse the route. On our journey together through the pages of this book we shall start at Elizabeth as it is known today, or Elizabethtown, as it was called in the seventeenth century.

Today the eastern end of the road is an unattractive industrial area on Newark Bay with nothing left of the original ferry. The actual site of the ferry is marked by the rotting piles of a later dock. It was here, at the end of present-day Elizabeth Avenue in Elizabethport, that the early sail ferries departed for Manhattan as far back as 1679. Here also, General Washington and his wife stepped down from their coach

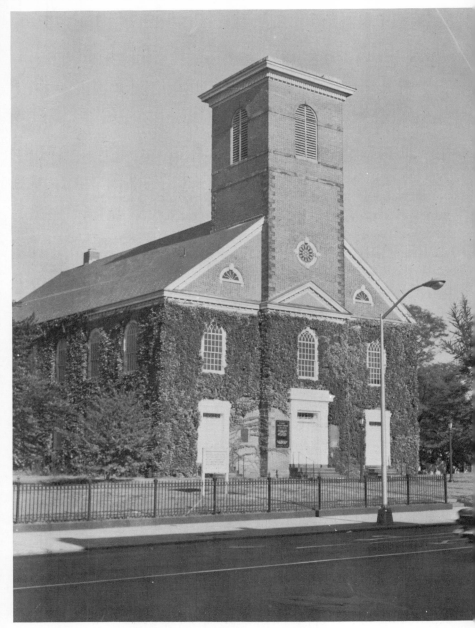

The Old First Church in Elizabeth.

on their journey from Mount Vernon to New York in 1789. At the ferry they boarded a gaily decorated barge which carried them to the Battery in Manhattan for Washington's inauguration as the first President of the United States.

Present-day Elizabeth is a city with a great historic heritage and Old First Church and the churchyard beside it are indeed hallowed ground. It was in the original building that the General Assembly met from 1666 to 1682. The present building was erected in 1789 and, except for the lack of the former tall steeple, it remains today about as it was nearly two centuries ago. The city also bears the distinction of being the oldest English-speaking community in New Jersey and Old First Church was the first in which services were conducted in English. During the Colonial and early Federal periods Elizabeth had a large and active group of the Sons of Liberty and other patriotic organizations and many descendants of the members still observe and cherish the distinctive past of their city.

Boxwood Hall, on East Jersey Street, was the home of Elias Boudinot, the first President of the Continental Congress. Later, he introduced the resolution in the U.S. House of Representatives that caused President Washington to proclaim November 26, 1789, our first Thanksgiving Day. After the murder of Parson Caldwell at Elizabethtown Point his body was thrown on the steps of Boudinot Hall. The British intended it as a warning to the American patriots, but after hearing the fiery speech delivered by Boudinot, while standing over the Parson's body, the Patriots were more determined than ever to get rid of British rule.

Just beyond the northern boundary of the city still stands Liberty Hall which was built in 1773 by William Livingston, the first Governor of the State of New Jersey. It was in this

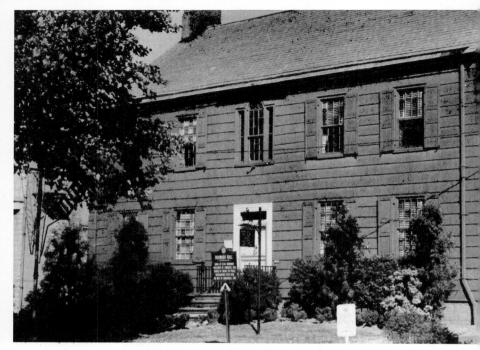

Boxwood Hall in Elizabeth.

house that Sally, the Governor's daughter, married John Jay, who later became the First Chief Justice of the United States. The Washingtons, Alexander Hamilton, the Marquis de Lafayette and many other illustrious people of the Colonial period were frequent guests here.

Where the Public Library now stands, on the corner of Broad Street and Rahway Avenue, the latter the Old York Road, formerly stood several famous stage taverns. Among them were the Indian Queen and Cornelisse's.

Much of the original route of our road from Elizabeth to Westfield is lost today in a maze of streets and highways. Therefore the next point of interest on our journey will be Westfield's historic Presbyterian Church. The first log church, which stood near the site of the present building, was erected

90

in 1735. The present church was built in 1861. The bell from an earlier church that was rung to warn the Patriots of the approach of the British hangs in the belfry of the present building. The earlier church was the scene of the trial and conviction of James Morgan, a British soldier who was hanged at "Gallows Hill" on North Broad Street. It was Morgan who murdered "Fighting Parson" Caldwell in Elizabethtown.

In 1684 some Scottish immigrants, who had landed at Perth Amboy, followed an Indian path north toward the Watchung hills, looking for a place to settle. They found a location to their liking and so they decided to make that area their home. The only possessions they could bring with them were the tools, seeds, and other things that could be carried on their backs. Thus the present-day Scotch Plains came into being.

The path those settlers used to travel north was bisected at the settlement by an east-west Indian path at the place where the immigrants settled. This path later became a part of the Old York Road.

The old tavern that is still standing on Front Street served travelers on the Old York Road for a century or more. The center part of the present building dates back to 1737. This venerable building has been continuously occupied, either as an inn or as a residence, since it was built. Surrounding the tavern today are several shops of Colonial design that add to the charm of the place.

Continuing our journey west on Front Street to and through Plainfield, we are still following approximately the original stage route. Depending upon the old map or text source consulted, there seem to be some divergent opinions about the course of the road from Plainfield west to Bound Brook. Old maps show the road going to New Market after leaving Plainfield, and we believe much of the confusion is due to the fact that New Market, or Quibbletown, as it was sometimes known, embraced much of what is now Dunellen. Therefore, it seems reasonable to assume that the road did in fact continue north of the tracks of the Central of New Jersey Railroad, on about the path of present day Main Street to and through to the west end of that community, then through present-day Middlesex Borough to Bound Brook.

Before leaving Plainfield, however, let us stop for a bit and see the Friends Meeting House on Watchung Avenue which was built in 1788. We should also visit the Nathaniel Drake House, now a museum, on West Front Street, which

Friends Meetinghouse in Plainfield.

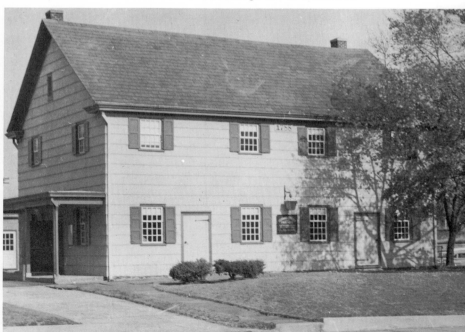

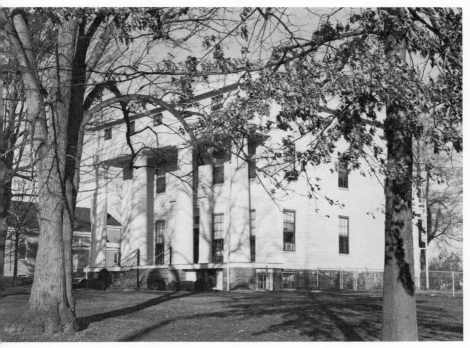

Duncan Phyfe House near Dunellen, now used as a church school.

was used by Washington as a meeting place with his scouts and spies.

As in the vicinity of Elizabeth, our original road here is lost in the network of present streets and highways so it is necessary to drive on to Dunellen. Before continuing through Dunellen we should turn left and drive down New Market Road to see the Duncan Phyfe House. This beautiful building in the Classic Revival style, with its imposing columns, is one of the finest buildings of that architectural style in the country. Duncan Phyfe, the world-renowned furniture craftsman, built the house for his daughter Eliza in 1814. Phyfe was famous as a cabinetmaker and his early nineteenth-century work was influenced by French Empire style and the designs of Sheraton and of Hope. We well remember, many

93

years ago, his workshop in the rear of the house and, when we last saw it shavings still covered the floor. They were possibly the last he made before his death.

A left turn at the west end of Dunellen will take us to and through the village of Lincoln, a part of Middlesex Borough. The main street and highway to Bound Brook follows approximately the original route of the Old York Road. Crossing the Bound Brook, which is the eastern boundary line of the borough, we are again in a community with a great historic heritage. Bound Brook was, in fact, the first settlement in Somerset County.

At the eastern end of the borough a left turn through the railroad underpass brings us to a piece of the original Old York Road. Near the Raritan River and between the tracks of the Lehigh Valley and the Central of New Jersey is an old stone bridge that dates back to the seventeenth century. It was to the east of this bridge that the Old York Road left the King's Highway it had followed from the forks of the Raritan, and continued north and east to its terminous at Elizabethtown. The tracks of the Central Railroad of New Jersey were laid near the route of our road from Bound Brook west to Somerville.

The first house in Bound Brook was erected in 1683 by Thomas Codrington. The house, of which no trace remains, was built on an elevated site said to have been an Indian burying ground, and this is the origin of the legend that the house was haunted. So strong was this belief, during the early years of the dwelling, that the servants dared not go out alone at night for fear they would be carried away by an Indian ghost. The house stood for over one hundred and seventy years until it was torn down in 1854. It was known as "Racawachanna," an Indian name meaning, "the loamy flats by the running brook."

Near the Middlebrook, the west boundary of the borough, formerly stood the Fisher Tavern. It is said that the first Masonic Lodge in Somerset County was organized here. Whether or not that is true, it is a fact that General Washington did attend Masonic meetings in the Tavern, which was a favorite of both officers and enlisted men of the Continental Army.

On the south face of First Watchung Mountain is Camp Middlebrook. According to tradition, the thirteen-star flag, reputedly made by Betsy Ross of Philadelphia, was first raised over American troops there. Even the Washington Camp Ground Association, which in 1889 dedicated the site as a historic memorial, believed the story about the flag, as is indicated on a plaque at the Camp Ground, which is inscribed, "On this spot the stars and stripes were first unfurled over the Continental Army after their official adoption by Congress June 14, 1777. By authority of Congress the Betsy Ross flag flies here twenty-four hours a day."

We are reluctant to admit that our cherished beliefs over the years about the flag must be drastically revised in the interest of historical accuracy.

On June 14, 1777, Congress did in fact pass the resolution: RESOLVED: that the flag of the United States be made of thirteen stripes, alternate red and white; that the union be thirteen stars, white in a blue field, representing a new constellation. However, further research has not uncovered any evidence that the so-called Betsy Ross flag was delivered to General Washington at Camp Middlebrook, or, in fact, that Betsy Ross made such a flag during the time the Army was at Middlebrook.

For those who would like to separate the myths from the facts about our flag we would recommend the reading of a recent book, *The History of the United States Flag,* by Milo M. Quaife, Melvin J. Weig, and Roy E. Appleman.

Just west of the Middlebrook still stands the Philip Van Horn Mansion. During the Revolution this beautiful Colonial house, with its long lane leading down to the Old York Road, was a New Jersey landmark. Its one-time beauty gradually deteriorated and it seemed that this lovely reminder of Colonial times was likely to become a complete ruin. However, the American Cyanamid Company, the present owner of the property, has restored the house and it is now used as an employees' club.

Few of the eighteenth-century houses have a more interesting background than does "Phil's Hill," or "Convivial Hall," as the Van Horn House was better known. During the Revolution, Van Horn, whose sympathies were with the Crown, remained a neutral during the war, and he entertained both British and American officers lavishly. His five lovely daughteres were perhaps among the main attractions to the officers of both armies. Two of the daughters later married American officers.

Many interesting stories have been told over the years about this famous place. One is that General Richard Henry Lee, known as Light Horse Harry, during one of the entertainments, rode his horse through the wide entrance hall and up the grand stairway to the second floor. Convivial Hall, indeed! There is another story that seems hard to believe about Lord Cornwallis and General Benjamin Lincoln of the Continentals. It is said that on the morning of the battle of Bound Brook, April 13, 1777, Lord Cornwallis had breakfast in the Van Horn House and that having withdrawn his forces and hidden in the nearby woods all day, General Lincoln of the American Army enjoyed dinner there.

Continuing west over the Bound Brook-Somerville road from the Van Horn house about two miles, a left turn is made to visit the site of the old Dutch Church, which was burned by Colonel John Graves Simcoe's raiders. Just before reaching the Raritan River a state marker tells of the former church location and, across the road and a few hundred yards in from the road, may be found the Van Veghten House, on a bluff above the Raritan. This charming old house, built near the beginning of the eighteenth century, is occupied by a tenant farmer, one of many who have tilled this land for over two hundred years. The house was old when the Old York Road first passed it. Washington and

The Van Veghten House at Finderne, General Nathanael Greene's headquarters during the Middlebrook encampment.

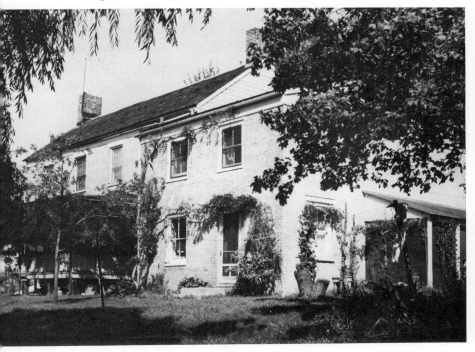

his army marched by on their way from their victory at Princeton in January to winter quarters at Morristown.

It was here that the famous Christmas party, given by General and Mrs. Greene for General and Mrs. Washington, was held. At this party Alexander Hamilton met the lovely Betsy Schuyler whom he later married at her home in Morristown.

To stand today near this venerable place, particularly on a quiet spring or summer day, viewing the wide sweep of the Raritan to the west and to the east, and the beautiful countryside around it, one finds it easy to understand why the Dutch settlers, who had come to the Raritan Valley from as far away as Albany, called this valley "the pleasantest and best inhabited land that man can behold."

Returning to the Bound Brook-Somerville road, we next enter Somerville and the first place of interest is the modern Somerset Hotel on the right side of Main Street. The present-day structure is on the former location of the famous stage stop that was known as Tunison's Tavern. Some authorities believe that part of the original tavern is incorporated within the present building. Tunison's was considered one of the best between the Hudson and the Delaware. Like most taverns of its time, it was a popular meeting place for local residents who frequented the place to get news of other places from the travelers over the stage road.

There was an earlier tavern than Tunison's that formerly stood at the forks of the road at the western end of the town, which at that time was called Raritan. The stages of the Swift-Sure Line regularly stopped there.

All of what is now the two communities of Raritan and Somerville was, until the beginning of the nineteenth century, known as Raritan. When the county seat was moved there from Millstone in 1814, the borough of Somerville was created.

From an advertisement that appeared in the Somerset County *Messenger* in 1826, the town was described as follows: "The village of Somerville combines many advantages. It is central, healthy, pleasant and easy of access. The Swift-Sure stage from New York to Philadelphia passes through three times a week, and a stage connecting itself with a line of stages and steamboats at New Brunswick, leaves the village every morning for that city and returns in the afternoon."

Our route continues along Main Street and under the railroad underpass. A left turn on Middagh Street takes us to the Old Dutch Parsonage and just beyond is the Wallace House, or Washington's Headquarters as it is better known. George and Martha Washington lived in this house and used it as a military headquarters on several occasions during the years 1778-79. It was here that Washington planned the strategy for the Indian campaign, that, successfully executed under Generals John Sullivan and James Clinton, broke the power of the Iroquois, the Six Nations who were the powerful British allies.

The Headquarters, formerly owned by the Revolutionary Memorial Society and now maintained as a historic site by the State of New Jersey, is open to the public for a very small fee.

Many of the original furnishings have been returned and one piece especially, a rare grandfather's clock which stands on the stair landing, has an interesting history. At one time when the village was threatened by the British, the works of the clock were sealed in a waterproof box and buried in the nearby river. The clock is at least two hundred years old and still keeps good time. On the second floor is a nine-foot box

99

that was General Washington's personal trunk which, when traveling, was placed on a wheeled carrier and pulled along the road by a mule.

During the occupation of the house by the Washingtons many of the General's aides and officers were frequent visitors and overnight guests. Among them were the Marquis de Lafayette, William Colfax, General Sullivan, Lord Stirling, and many others. Conrad Alexandre Gérard, the first ambassador of France to the American Colonies, was also a guest on several occasions.

It is said that the Wallace House was selected as a headquarters because of its convenience to Camp Middlebrook and to the quarters of many of the high-ranking officers who met with the General to discuss plans and strategy. General Greene was quartered at the Van Veghten house at Finderne, Baron von Steuben at the Staats House at South Bound Brook. Other staff officers within a few miles' radius could be quickly notified of meetings by the fast-riding couriers who were constantly on the Old York Road.

Across the street from the Headquarters is the Old Dutch Parsonage, which was built by the Reverend John Frelinghuysen in 1751. He and his family were among the earliest of the Dutch settlers in the valley. Ministers, statesmen, and military officers have added to the luster of this family over the years, and descendants of the Reverend John are still contributing to the public service in Congress and in other important offices.

The Parsonage is now owned by the local chapter of the Daughters of the American Revolution who maintain it as a museum, open to the public at certain hours. It was in this building that the first theological seminary of the Dutch

Reformed Church was instituted. This later became Rutgers College, now Rutgers, The State University.

Adjoining Somerville on the west is the borough of Raritan and it is west of this community that a journey over the Old York Road will be most rewarding. Except for some new houses, the countryside appears much as it has for the past century. In fact, it was only twenty-five or so years ago that much of our road west of the Raritan was a high-crowned dirt road, as it had been since it was opened in 1764.

At the west end of the town there is a monument commemorating the friendly relations with the Indians that made possible the widening of the Indian path into the Kings Highway which later became a part of the Old York Road.

To the left of the road, as one travels west, is the canal originally built to supply power for the turbines that generated electricity for the fabulous James B. Duke estate across the river. The canal and the land as far as the juncture of the South and North Branches of the Raritan is now a part of the Somerset County park system. The Indian name for the meeting place of the North and South Branch rivers was "Tucca-Ramma-Hacking" which meant the "meeting place of the waters."

The early settlers of the Raritan Valley were mainly the Dutch from New York City, Long Island, and, in fact, from as far away as Albany. They drove their great wagons, piled high with all their worldly goods, over the Old Dutch Road from Elizabethtown to New Brunswick and then up the Kings Highway to Bound Brook and on to the forks of the river.

The wagons, drawn by four and sometimes six draft horses, with the Dutch families dressed in their quaint costumes, created a great deal of interest as they passed along the road.

Tunison's Tavern in Somerville was a favorite overnight stop, and in the evening the travelers from New York would visit there with the local people to exchange news for suggestions as to the best places to settle. They conversed in the common language, Dutch, as English was seldom heard in the valley during those early days.

What were the thoughts of those sturdy Dutch people as they made their way slowly through the Raritan Valley? We cannot know, of course, but we can understand something of their joy and satisfaction in knowing that soon they would establish a home in the lush and lovely valley, on land as fertile as any they had known in the old country.

The Raritan River, the name of which was derived from the Indian designation "Laleton," meaning "forked river," ran through the heart of the valley and provided a plentiful supply of water for the cattle and the many grist mills that were built along its shores. The Dutch soon learned, as the Indians had known for centuries, that the spring freshets deposited a new layer of rich river loam on the meadows each year. Bountiful crops were harvested on the meadows. The grains were later ground in the nearby mills and the flour floated down river in flatboats to tidewater at what is now Landing Bridge, above New Brunswick.

As far back as 1683, Thomas Rudyard, in his book on the American Colonies, mentioned the Raritan as a river that would probably assume large importance in the commerce of the Colonies. Peter Kalm, a visiting Swedish scholar, in his book of impressions of this country, said that the Raritan would one day be the chief waterway in America. He was right at least in his prediction of the importance of the river to the economy of New Jersey.

In 1806, John Davis, an English poet, described this lovely stream in his "Ode to the Raritan, Queen of Rivers":

> All thy wat'ry face
> Reflected with a purer grace,
> Thy many turnings through the trees,
> Thy bitter journey to the seas,
> Thou queen of Rivers, Raritan.

The great movement to settle the Raritan Valley during the latter part of the seventeenth century and the early years of the eighteenth century was partly a result of the publication of an enthusiastic report made public in Holland by Cornelius van Tierhoven about the farming possibilities of the valley. He reported that the district was inhabited by a nation called the "Raritangs" who lived on a fresh-water stream that flowed through the center of a lowland which the Indians cultivated. As most of the state was forested, the meadows appealed to the Dutch because it would be easy to farm them without the labor of clearing the land of trees as was necessary with most interior land tracts.

From the forks west to the Delaware the lovely rolling countryside of Somerset and Hunterdon Counties and the many eighteenth-century buildings, most of which have been standing since, and in many cases, before the Old York Road was opened, are vivid reminders of an earlier day and a simpler way of life. Side roads with names like "Barley" and "Wheat Sheaf" add to the charm of this part of the road. From this point west to the Delaware, and in fact all the way to Philadelphia, one sees the street and highway signs reading "Old York Road."

From the forks the present-day road follows very closely

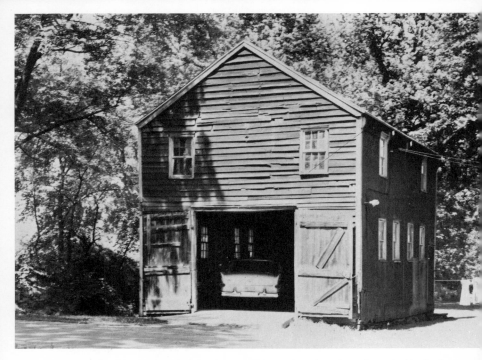

The blacksmith shop at Centerville, believed to have been built during the latter part of the eighteenth century.

the route of the original road, except where bends have been straightened out. It runs due west with a sharp left turn at a point near Readington, which during the earlier days was known as Readings. To follow the road to Centerville the modern Highway 202 is crossed twice. It is only a few miles to this lovely village, little changed from the days when it was the overnight stop on the stage road between New York and Philadelphia. It is a place that one should not hurry through. The tavern, for many years the overnight stop, was burned down but much of the original horse barn is still standing. It is now a community center. The center of the village is a crossroads, with the old store on one corner and the site of the former tavern on another. The old blacksmith shop is across the road from the store and is now used as a private garage. Not far west of the store, now a private residence, is a tiny building that was a barber shop many years ago.

The most interesting building is of course the barn where the relief horses were stabled during the days of the stagecoach. There is some question as to just how much of the present building is original but it appears that most of the timber frame is. The siding, which was originally plain barn boards, has been covered with shingles to keep the weather out and make possible the use of the barn for community affairs.

No more, as it was stated in a vivid description in "Two-Hundred and Fifty Years of Somerset," can "the blare of a coach horn be heard a half mile away, as the east- or west-bound coach approached the village of Centerville. The four or six horses a-lather and the green and gold coach flashing and swaying as it came round the bend was a wonderful sight to behold. The coachman, riding aloft, resplendent in buckskin breeches, top boots, red vest, and gold-banded silk hat. With the driver cracking his whip, the stage would swing into the inn yard with a flourish."

The present-day residents of Centerville have a deep sense of history and they are proud that their village remains a quiet oasis in the turbulent and uncertain world of today. Fortunately, the modern highway is far enough away to divert most of the motor traffic. We sincerely hope that the quiet charm of this little village will endure for a long time to come.

The small stream that runs through the village was the site of former Indian villages. Many evidences of their earlier occupation have been found along its banks.

There are few villages like Centerville left today. Here and there in some parts of New England one may still be found. The authors find such places a source of renewal, and in them feel the pull of events of an earlier day. It is good to feel such things, we believe, when so many changes are taking place in the world around us. When visiting Centerville, particularly on a quiet summer day, as we have done so many times, stop a while and just listen. One can almost believe that the horn of an approaching stage can be heard.

Three Bridges, a few miles west of Centerville, is still the quiet little hamlet it has always been and a few miles beyond is Reaville where our road meets the Amwell Road to New Brunswick. The Old York Road makes a sharp right turn and continues west to Larison's Corner, or Pleasant Corners as it was also known.

When the Swift-Sure Stage Line first opened for business between Philadelphia and Elizabethtown Point in 1769 it followed the Old York Road between Three Bridges, Reaville, and Ringoes. However, at around the beginning of the nineteenth century the stage route was shifted from the Old York Road at Ringoes and continued to Flemington for the overnight stop. From that point it continued to Centerville. We shall, in our journey, follow the original route.

From Reaville the road runs along a high ridge and the beautiful countryside is visible for miles. As Larison's Corner is reached, the village church is on the left with the cemetery across the road. Here are buried several generations of the early settlers of the area, who for the most part were of German ancestry. Across from the cemetery formerly stood Larison's Tavern, described in detail earlier in these pages.

Just west of Larison's Corner is Ringoes, which was settled about 1721. This was a very important community dur-

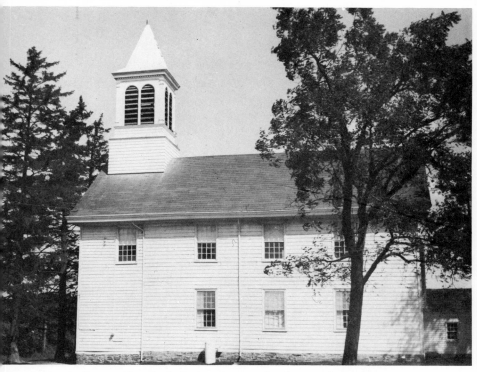

Larison's Corner Church, built in 1817, replaced a previous structure built in 1749. In the present congregation are many descendants of early settlers of the area.

ing the days of the first settlement of the Amwell Valley, with the village the trading center for miles around.

In the center of the village still stands the Jersey sandstone building that was the Amwell Academy, but which is now unfortunately a package store. The Academy was not built until 1811 and when it opened it became very popular as an educational institution, attracting students from as far away as Baltimore.

Beyond the Academy on the left side of the road is the Landis house, believed to be one of the oldest standing buildings in Hunterdon County. It was here that Major General

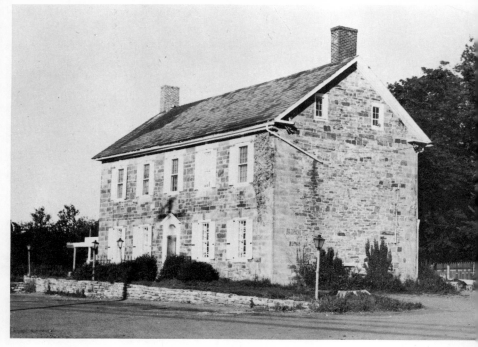

Amwell Academy at Ringoes.

the Marquis de Lafayette was brought from Valley Forge by a local doctor to recuperate from an illness. The house is often referred to as the Lafayette House. The original beauty of the sandstone walls of this Dutch architecture has been hidden with plaster, and concrete columns now adorn the front porch.

Ringoes has an interesting history dating back to the first land purchase near the beginning of the eighteenth century. The first building was a log tavern, also used as a residence, at the junction of the roads to Lambertville, then known as Coryell's Ferry and present-day Route 69, a former Indian path to Trenton. The latter was described as "one running north and south, being the path of the Minsie Indians, from

Muskanecum Hills to the wigwams of the Assunpinks [Trenton]." The Lambertville road was the "great east and west path" (the Naraticong Indian path) which was later to become a part of the Old York Road.

Soon after Ringo built his cabin tavern, other settlers bought land in the valley and built their homes. Many of those early houses are still occupied by the descendants of the first settlers. One of the oldest houses is that built by Peter Fisher on land he purchased in 1729. His first home was a log cabin and the present house was not built until 1741.

Peter Fisher and his friend Peter Johann Rockefeller came to this country on a sailing ship from Germany. Their ship was bound for New York but was blown off course and landed its passengers in Philadelphia. Peter Fisher and his

The Landis House at Ringoes as it appeared during the nineteenth century.

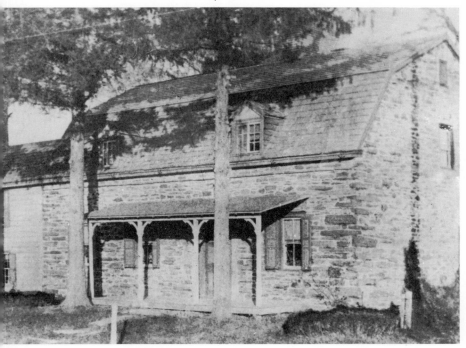

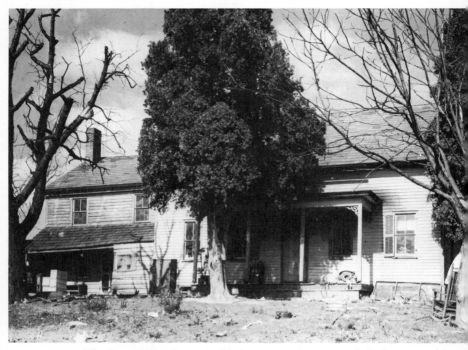

The Peter Fisher homestead before restoration. It was built in 1741 with timber rafted down the Delaware.

friend walked up the Delaware Valley intending to walk overland to New York, their original destination, but when they saw the country of western Hunterdon they decided to settle there. Accordingly, they bought adjoining farms west of Ringoes and near Rocktown.

The authors owned, until a few years ago when it was stolen, the original deed to the land that was conveyed to Peter Fisher from Benjamin Field in 1729. The deed was also signed with the mark of Indian Chief Himhammoe.

Jacob Fisher, a grandson of Peter, built a stone house on the Old York Road a mile east of Lambertville, as it is known today. He was a blacksmith by trade and conducted a smithy in which he made axes, chisels, knives, and other implements that in that day could only be obtained from a blacksmith. Until the latter part of the eighteenth century there were no industrial establishments for the manufacture of such things as tools and implements.

Dr. C. W. Larison, who married one of the granddaughters of Peter Fisher, was a well-known figure in the field of education during the middle of the nineteenth century in Ringoes. He purchased the Amwell Academy about 1868. Among his many contributions was his efforts to establish phonetic spelling. In 1883 he wrote and published a book entitled "Fonic Speler and Sylabater" and on the title page of his book was the statement that it was "Desind As an Ad in Aquiring A Noleg Ov The Fundamental Principls Ov the English Lanwag."

The right fork of the road out of Ringoes to the west is the Old York Road. In one or two places the present road

Fireplace in the Fisher homestead.

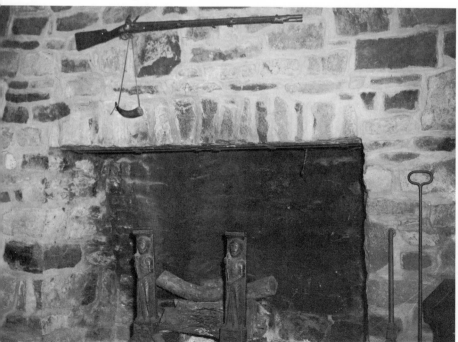

leaves the original route; otherwise, Route 202 from Ringoes to Lambertville follows the same path as it did when it became the Old York Road in 1764.

On the right, a half-mile west of Ringoes is the Skillman House, generally known as the "Queen of the Valley." At either end of this impressive brick Colonial mansion are massive chimney breasts. In several of the rooms there are some of the finest examples of hand-carved fireplace mantles to be found anywhere. Some of the paneling is beautifully tinted from age and the wide floor boards are original. It is said that the brick of which the house was made was molded on the farm. The hand-carved dentil work under the eaves is exquisite. The cellar floor is paved with brick, as in many houses of that period, to provide a cool place for perishables.

The Skillman homestead on the Old York Road a mile southwest of Ringoes.

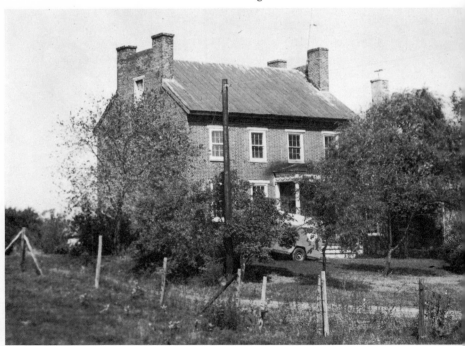

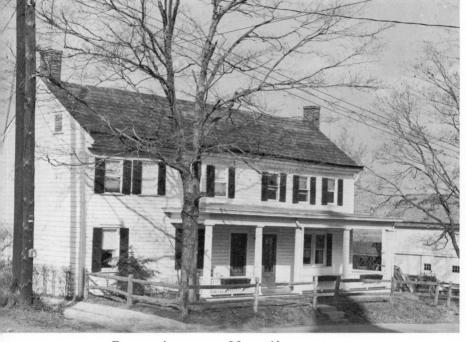

Former stage tavern at Mount Airy.

From this point the hills of the Delaware Valley are in sight. About half way to Lambertville the original route makes a wide swing to the left from the main road, and passes through the hamlet of Mt. Airy. In the center of the village still stands the old sandstone community building that was the Holcombe storehouse, built in the middle of the eighteenth century. It was a common storehouse for the farmers for miles around who stored their flax, grain, tallow, and other farm products until they could be carted over the road to Coryell's Ferry and floated down river in the Durham boats during the spring high water.

In view of the fact that there were very few roads other than the local "ways" in and between villages, those who were able to store their produce in the Mt. Airy storehouse were fortunate. The Delaware River was their highway to a good income.

Two of the early stage taverns are still standing in Mt. Airy. Both are now used as private residences. The old church and churchyard are interesting and worth a visit.

Just a short distance west of the village the old road again merges with the present highway. As the road drops into the town of Lambertville, one's sense of history is sharpened. A drive down along the river and a short walk enables the tourist to get a close look at the canal feeder and the old lock and locktender's house. The house is shaded in summer by huge old sycamore trees and the light and shadow effect on a sunny day makes the scene a favorite with artists and photographers. It is well worth seeing even though the lock gates no longer function. Concrete spillways now regulate the

The Delaware and Raritan Canal feeder below Lambertville.

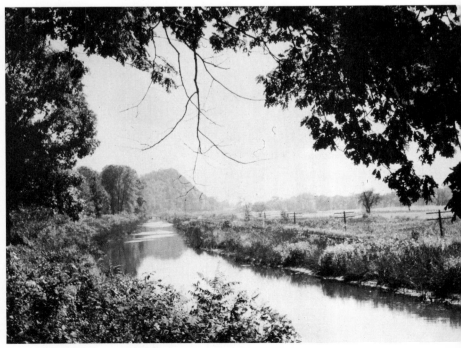

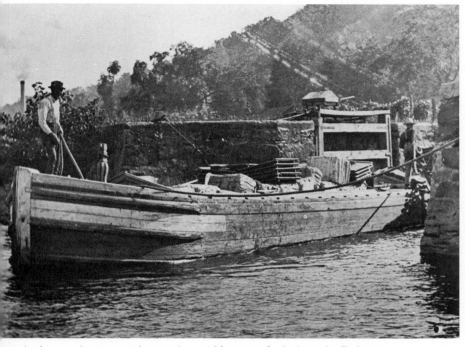

A nineteenth-century picture of a canal barge at the lock on the Delaware and Raritan Canal feeder at Lambertville.

flow of the water. The feeder was built in 1832 to carry water from the Delaware River to the main Delaware and Raritan Canal at Trenton. In those days there was no mechanical earth-moving equipment and the feeder and the canal were built with pick, shovel, and horse-drawn drags. The labor for that tremendous job was largely drawn from the ranks of Irish immigrants. During the course of the construction, an epidemic of Asiatic cholera broke out, and many of the laborers who died from it were buried along the banks of the waterway.

The job was finally finished and both the feeder and the canal were ready for navigation in the summer of 1834. The water of the feeder, which flowed to the canal by gravity from

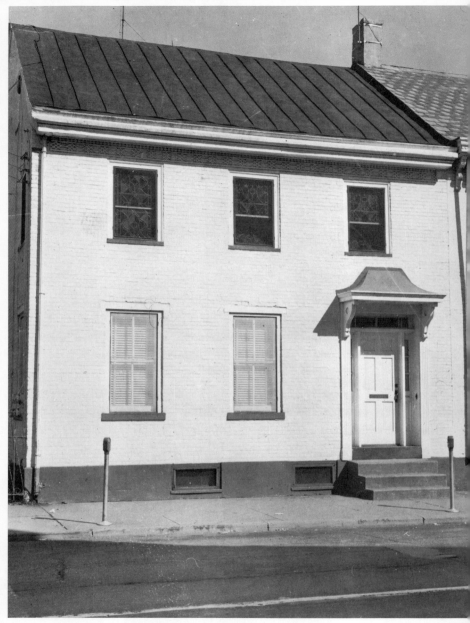

The home of James Marshall's parents on Bridge Street in Lambertville.

the higher elevation at the source in the Delaware, kept the forty-four miles of the canal from New Brunswick to Bordentown supplied with water, as it does the canal from Trenton to New Brunswick today.

Lambertville has many historic places. On the north side of Bridge Street stands the James Philip Marshall house. It was here in his father's house that James Wilson Marshall was born in 1810. Young Marshall was a carpenter and he worked his way west until he reached Kansas where he joined a wagon train bound for California. While building a sawmill on the American River, he was the first to discover gold, thus starting the famous gold rush of 1849. Marshall and his partner, General John Sutter, became famous but both died penniless.

Farther west on Bridge Street is the historic Lambertville House, built by Captain John Lambert in 1812, two years before the first covered bridge was built across the Delaware at that point. This quaint hostelry is little changed from the days when it first served travelers over the Old York Road, which passes its doors. Modern conveniences have been added but it still has the charm of an old inn. Jack Allen conducts the hotel as did earlier hosts and, for those who enjoy an overnight stop in an old inn and exceptionally good food, the Lambertville House is highly recommended by the authors, who have often been guests there.

In the churchyard of the nearby Presbyterian Church is the grave of George Coryell, the son of Emanuel who founded the village of Coryell's Ferry which is now Lambertville. On the marker over the grave is inscribed the following: "Here lies the body of George Coryell, who died February 18, 1851, aged ninety-one years." On the reverse

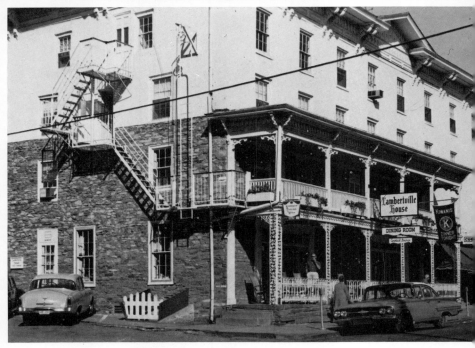

The Lambertville House, built in 1812, replaced an earlier stone tavern.

side is chiseled, "The last survivor of the six men who laid the Father of our Country in his tomb."

Up the road toward Stockton, near the north boundary of the village, is the Richard Holcombe House in which General Washington was a guest on two occasions.

While Lambertville does not seem to appeal to tourists as much as does her neighbor New Hope across the river, it is less hectic and the charm of its many historic sites, antique shops, book stores, and good places to dine may be more quietly enjoyed.

From Lambertville to Stockton and the country inland toward Flemington more and more people of the arts are settling as permanent residents. For the lover of antiques the whole area is a happy hunting ground. The summer stock season attracts thousands nightly to both the Bucks County Playhouse in New Hope and to the Music Circus on the hill above Lambertville.

James P. Snell in his *History of Hunterdon and Somerset Counties* said of Lambertville, "The hills immediately to the east and southeast of the town are quite bold and abrupt, but those to the northeast and north rise up with gentle acclivity. From these hills there are extensive and beautiful views of the surrounding country.

"From the most elevated points near the town may be seen the range of the Orange Mountain, nearly 30 miles away, Pickel's Mountain, near White House station, in the upper part of this county and distant about 25 miles, and, about the same distance to the northwest, the Haycock Mountain, in Pennsylvania. Few places have more picturesque surroundings than has Lambertville, and the wonder is that it has not attracted more of the attention of the lovers of fine scenery."

Since Snell wrote his description in 1880, many people have come to love the beauty of the hills and the river valley in the vicinity of Lambertville.

John Holcombe of Abington, Pennsylvania, purchased a large tract of land in this part of the province in 1705 when the entire area was a wilderness crossed only by a few Indian paths. One of those was a path from Neshaminy, in Pennsylvania, to the Indian encampments along the Raritan. The combination of heavy forest along the river and the river itself made this place a favorite haunt of fish and game. The last wolf was killed in this vicinity in 1880.

Many people still living remember the great shad runs up the Delaware River in former years. It is said that in a single day as many as twenty-five hundred shad would be caught by local fishermen. During the height of the run they were actually scooped up in bushel baskets.

Driving over the iron bridge to New Hope one may see on both sides of the river the former ferry landings which went out of business shortly after the first covered bridge was built.

Down the river a few miles, on the western shore, Bowman's Tower in Pennsylvania's Washington Crossing Park may be seen. It was the site of an important lookout during the Revolution and from it much of the Delaware Valley could be kept under observation.

Bucks County, Pennsylvania, attracts writers and artists generally. Some of the country's most famous are among the year-round residents there. They are naturally interested in the exceptional charm and beauty of the county. The facilities of Philadelphia are only an hour away and those of the New York City area are almost as close. Many from the county regularly commute to both those cities.

Today's visitor to New Hope finds a village where the atmosphere of an earlier century is combined with a bewildering array of shops, art exhibits, sculpture, and many similar places. The village is unique and travelers come from all over the country to visit and buy in the fascinating shops.

John Wells, the first settler, obtained a patent early in the eighteenth century on a grant of land of some one hundred acres to operate a ferry across the Delaware River. This was known as Wells' Ferry while the one across the river was called Coryell's Ferry. It must have been and is confusing as the name of Wells' Ferry was later changed to Coryell's Ferry. The community that rapidly grew up around the location of the early ferry, prospered as more and more mills were built on the little stream that entered the Delaware at that point.

The early ferryboats were small craft of many kinds. As early travel was on foot or on horseback, the passengers rode in the boat while the horse swam across the river behind it. Later, when wheeled vehicles came into general use, the ferries were larger, usually flatboats. They were equipped with hinged flaps at either end which, when lowered to the riverbank, enabled the driver to get his rig into the boat. Many early ferries were rowed and poled across the stream. Others, where it was possible to string a cable across from which the ferry was attached with a pulley arrangement, used the current as a means of propulsion.

Until a few years ago, on the upper reaches of the Delaware River, several of the larger, vehicle-carrying flatboat ferries were still being operated. A few miles above New Hope one of the cable ferries is still being used to carry a Jeep across to an island.

One of the most interesting places in New Hope is Logan's Inn, built by John Wells in 1727 to serve the growing settlement and the travelers over the Old York Road. Originally the road passed down Ferry Street to the Ferry Landing. Later, in 1814, when the first covered bridge was built across the river, the stage route was changed to what is now Bridge Street and that became a part of our stage road. The Inn was named for James Logan who was William Penn's secretary. In the yard of the inn stands a metal cutout of an Indian with bow extended. It was erected to honor Chief

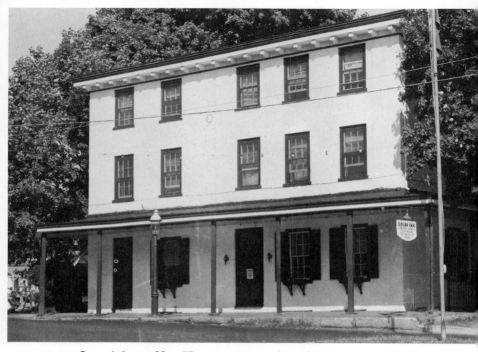

Logan's Inn at New Hope was a convenient place to stop for refreshments before taking the ferry to Lambertville.

Wingohocking of a local tribe who were very friendly with the early settlers. Later the Chief took Logan's name as a gesture of eternal friendship. Sometime near the end of the eighteenth century the Chief and his family moved to the Ohio frontier. There some renegade whites murdered his entire family. From that day on Chief Wingohocking, who had been so friendly with the white people, turned against them and waged savage warfare until he died in 1790.

Diagonally across Ferry Street from Logan's Inn is the stone building, now a public library, that was originally where ferry tolls were collected. This charming old structure, built early in the eighteenth century, is worth visiting and is open during library hours. The ground floor fireplace, then the only source of heat, is still used, and on a winter day when a wood fire is burning the smell of wood smoke is pleasant indeed. A narrow flight of stairs leads to the second floor and the original hand-hewn beams are mellowed with age.

Directly across Main Street from the Toll House stands the mansion built in 1784 by Benjamin Parry. It required three years to build and was considered one of the finest Colonial homes in Bucks County. Parry owned a mill across the river in New Jersey known as "The Prime Hope Mill." When that was destroyed by fire in 1790, a new mill was constructed on the Pennsylvania side of the river, on the site of present day Bucks County Playhouse. This mill was called "The New Hope Mill." Thus the village that was originally Wells' Ferry became New Hope, as it is today.

According to the *Pennsylvania Gazetteer*, New Hope was, in 1832, the largest manufacturing center in Bucks County.

Stone house in New Hope built by Benjamin Parry in 1784.

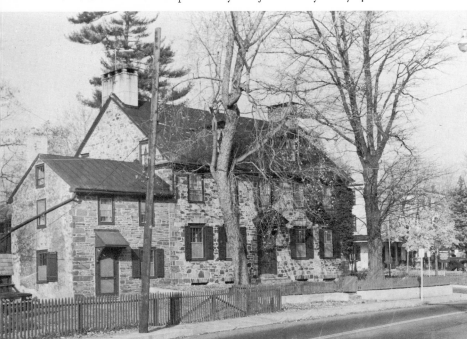

Today tourism is the most important business of the community.

As one drives or walks along Ferry Street today, the many attractive old buildings on both sides of the street are evidence of the fact that New Hope is a very old community. In fact it is the oldest in Solebury Township. Its beginning was a land grant in 1710 from William Penn.

While Washington Crossing Park, which begins a mile or so south of New Hope, is not actually a part of the story of the Old York Road, it is tied to our highway through the events of history.

Malta Island in the Delaware at the southern end of New Hope, has lost its original identity. It is now just a sand spit.

Although a detour from the Old York Road, we urge our readers to drive down along the river on Pennsylvania Route 32 and enjoy the many interesting places in this lovely park. It is only a few miles to the Thompson-Neely House. Nearby are the famous wild-flower gardens of the park. For those who wish to lunch in historic surroundings there are plenty of picnic spots. The river views, the canal beside the road, and the flanking hills, particularly Bowman's Hill, and many other features make this short detour very much worth while.

To delve a bit into Revolutionary history, visit the David Library of the American Revolution in the Memorial Building. The librarian, Mr. William Holland, is always gracious and welcomes interested visitors. An impressive collection of maps and original letters written by George Washington and other famous people of the Revolution may be inspected.

Returning to New Hope there are many interesting things to do; good places to dine and to shop; in summer a ride on

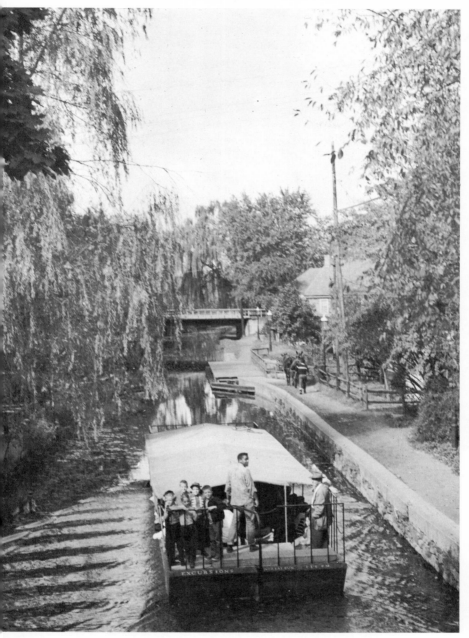

One of the summer attractions at New Hope is an hour's trip on a mule-
drawn barge along the Delaware Canal.

the mule-drawn canal barge, and the Bucks County Playhouse for an evening of the theater.

The jewel in the New Hope setting is the Delaware Canal which flows through the village. It was built in the middle of the nineteenth century to carry coal from the Lehigh area. The authors remember well the tiny coal barges that used the canal during the early part of this century. In fact, we could occasionally hitchhike on one of the string of barges and ride in our canoe without effort for a few miles. The bargeloads of coal destined for Philadelphia used the canal to its Delaware River terminous at Bristol. Those bound for New York were ferried across the Delaware above the wing dams and Wells' Falls and then continued down the canal feeder to the Delaware and Raritan Canal at Trenton. Coal was also carried by canal barge from Philipsburgh via the Morris and Essex Canal to the Hudson River at Jersey City.

The Delaware Canal, which is now a state park, is one of the loveliest recreational waterways in the country. As it passes through the countryside, it is today the setting not only for the older homes of an earlier century but many new ones. In New Hope, shops, homes and restaurants line its banks and add considerably to the charm of the village.

The authors, who have enjoyed the beauty of this waterway in many canoe journeys over the years, feel a special sense of gratitude to the members of the Delaware Valley Protective Association whose valiant efforts saved this historic waterway.

Those who have never seen a canal lock in operation may visit the restored lock at Lumberville. It is only seven miles north of New Hope. In the crisp fall weather a walk along

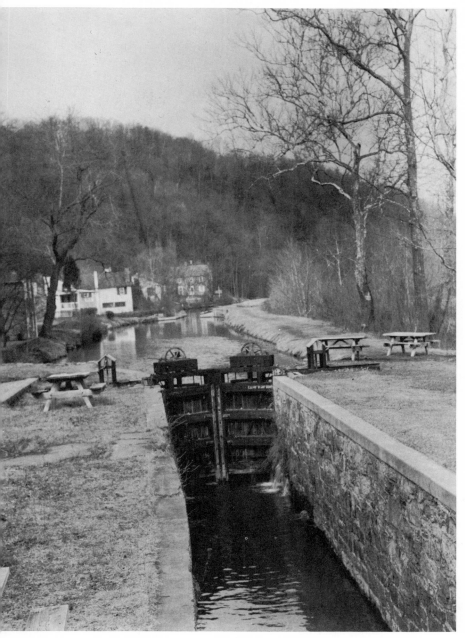

A lock on the Delaware Canal at Lumberville that has been restored to
operating condition.

the towpath is very worth while. While walking or for that matter, riding on the mule-drawn barge that is operated in the summer, the slow pace of travel gives one a better opportunity to contemplate the beauty and to recall the days of the operation of the canal.

Whether by car, canoe, mule barge, or walking, the entire canal is a joy to the artist and photographer with its mile after mile of beautiful scenery.

Driving west out of New Hope on Ferry Street our route merges with the present-day Pennsylvania Route 202, and follows it to a point just beyond the Solebury School on West Bridge Street. A street on the left, marked "The Old York Road," should be followed to continue the journey on the route of the original highway. This part of the road retains some of its original stone and plaster buildings and, at the point where Suggan Street crosses our road, a left turn takes the traveler to and across Aquetong Creek, on the bank of which may be seen the ruins of an early mill, now being restored. The mill was built by Richard Heath in 1702, and is believed to be the oldest one in Bucks County.

Returning to the Old York Road and turning left will enable the traveler to continue on the original route of the road for a few miles after which it again joins the present highway.

Among the many lovely pre-Revolutionary houses in this area is one that is known as Ingham Manor. Featured in Richard Pratt's *A Treasury of Early American Homes* it was described: "Built of what county people call 'tailored stone,' carefully cut and laid, its flat-arched windows and doorways, and its flanking wings at lower level, are signs of its pre-Revolutionary period, when stone houses began to replace the log cabins of the locality's earliest settlers." The

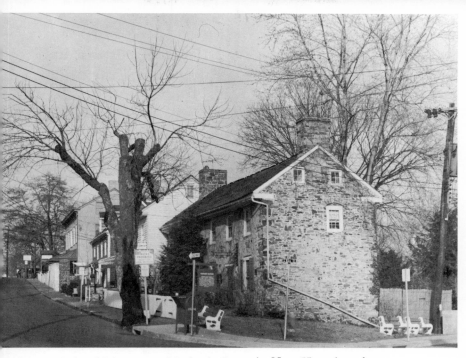

Many of the old houses on Mechanic Street in New Hope have been
converted to a variety of interesting shops.

book describes what was known as "the walk-in fireplace,"
the wide opening supported by a massive lintel log of oak.
A room such as this would have originally been the kitchen
and the winter livingroom. The floor of Pennsylvania tile
is typical, and the homespun Swedish table cover is set with
country ironstone. It is altogether possible that the pine
paneling of the livingroom at Ingham Manor is the work
of shipwrights who settled along the Delaware in the early
days, and who turned their hands to house carpentry when
boat building was slow.

West of Indian Spring, halfway up the hill on the right,
is another interesting house. It is called "Inghamdale," and
was probably built during the early eighteenth century.

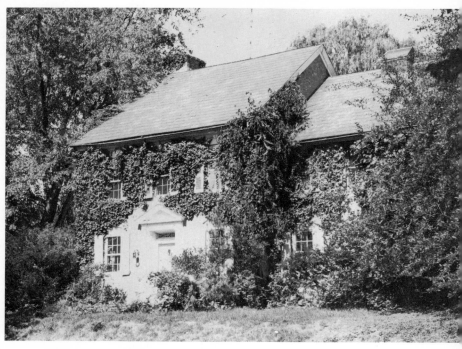

Inghamdale, one of the many eighteenth century houses along the
Pennsylvania section of the Old York Road.

Samuel D. Ingham, who was widely known as a statesman
and industrialist, was born there in 1779. He was Secretary
of the Treasury in Andrew Jackson's cabinet and held other
public offices. Ingham was a pioneer in the anthracite coal
industry and, as an ardent advocate of canals, was doubtless a
prime mover in the building of the Delaware Canal from
the Lehigh coal fields to Bristol.

Just east of Inghamdale, at Aquetong Cross Road, is a
pond of some sixteen acres that has been variously known
as "The Great Spring" and "Indian Spring." The Indians
knew it as "Aquetong," which meant "at the spring among
the bushes." Today, what appears to be a good-sized lake,
is actually a natural spring, said to be the largest between

Florida and Maine. It discharges over three million gallons of water a day. During the Colonial days it was the overflow from the spring that supplied the current in Aquetong Creek that turned the wheels of the many early mills along its banks.

Tedyuscung, the king of the Delaware Indians, was born near the spring and lived there with his braves. A rare degree of mutual respect existed between the white settlers and Tedyscung's people and they lived together in peace for many years.

Beyond the crossroad on the right may be seen another lovely stone house with an interesting history. It is the Paxton House, better known as "Rolling Green," built by Benjamin Paxton in 1748. During the Revolution, on several occasions, officers of the Continental Army were enter-

Aquetong, the Great Spring.

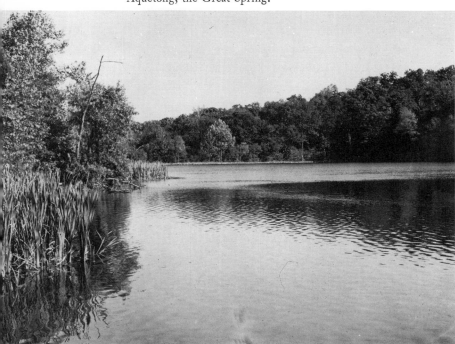

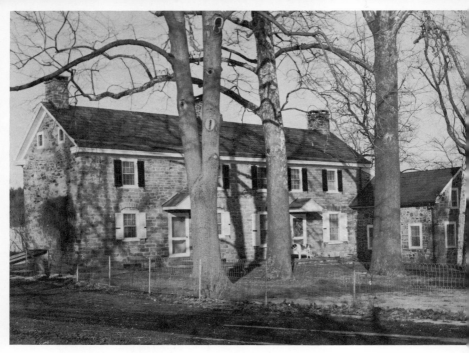

Rolling Green, where the Old York Road passes the Great Spring.

tained there. Like so many old houses, there are many stories of events said to have occurred in the place. One of those often-told tales was that on Christmas Eve, 1776, the night before the Delaware crossing, some Continental officers quartered in the house were cooking a Christmas meal of roast turkey and other traditional fixings. As they were about to enjoy the results of their efforts they received orders to march to the Delaware at McKonkey's Ferry. One can well imagine the disappointment of those officers but it is hoped that they received ample compensation in their glorious victory at Trenton two days later.

Just before entering Lahaska, one sees the buildings of Peddlers' Village a hundred yards in from the right side of the road. This complex of shops, including the Cock and Bull

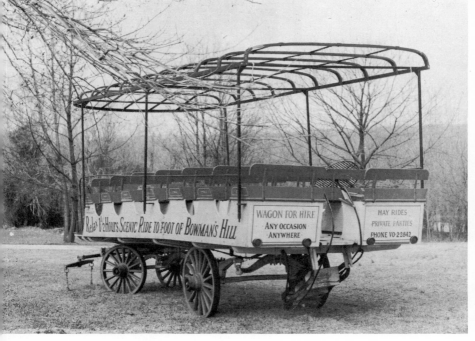

An old-time carryall at the Maple Grove Farm.

Restaurant, is a recent York Road tourist stop-over, operated by two young and energetic people, Sheila and Earl Jamison. The country shop called the "Hentown Country Store" and over twenty more shops displaying all kinds of quality merchandise attract visitors from all over the country.

Descending the hill out of Lahaska, a beautiful view of the Buckingham Valley unfolds. It was from this valley that Chief Isaac Still led the thirty or more members of the Delaware Tribe on their journey west to the Wabash in 1775. That small band was the last of the Lenni-Lenape to leave Pennsylvania. As Chief Still expressed it when they left the valley, "we are going far from war and rum." That small band of a once large and powerful nation that had lived in the area for centuries left, it is said, with their heads held

133

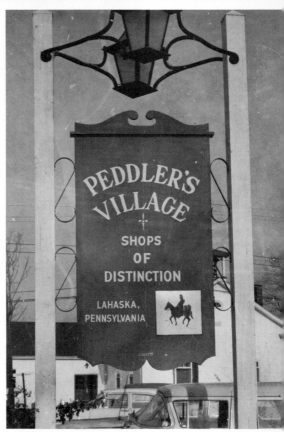

The Old York Road has its share of modern shopping centers and tourist attractions, in addition to the many historic sites along the way.

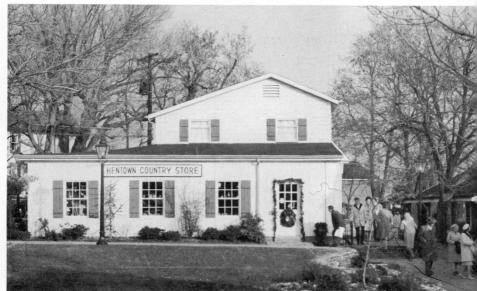

high. Perhaps also in their minds was the following lament, author unknown:

> Where is my home—my forest home?
> The proud land of my sires?
> Where stands the wigwam of my tribe?
> Where gleam the Council fires?
> Where are my fathers' hallowed graves?
> My friends so light and gay?
> Gone, gone forever from my view,
> Great Spirit, can it be?

Buckingham Mountain, about two hundred and fifty feet in height and about a thousand acres in extent, was the haunt of a notorious band of outlaws during the Revolution, known as the Doan boys, presumably brothers. Like the legends of most bands of outlaws, the telling of their deeds became larger as the tales were told and retold. Wolf Rocks, on top of the mountain, is near their former hideout.

Before the Civil War, the mountain was an underground station that sheltered slaves making their way to the north. As this is written, plans are being made by the Bucks County Commissioners to make the area a county park.

Beyond the crossroad on the right is the Quaker Meeting House and School. The present building was erected in 1768. The original log meetinghouse was in the cemetery and was built at the beginning of the eighteenth century. The open carriage sheds, still in use, appear today as they did a century ago. On the porch of the meetinghouse and outside on the grounds are stone "mounting" or "horseblocks," as they were known, used by the Friends to mount their horses or to enter the high farm wagons in which the families drove to services.

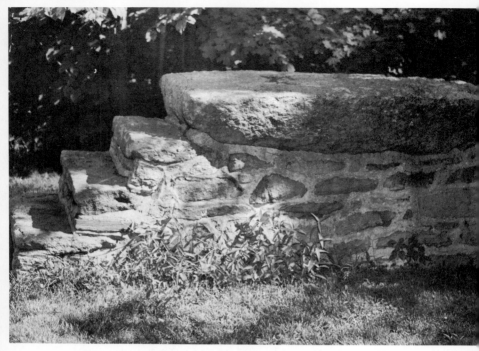

One of the mounting blocks on the grounds of the Friends Meetinghouse at Lahaska.

During the Revolution the meetinghouse was used as a hospital. Many of the soldiers who died there are buried in "The Strangers Plot."

At the Buckingham crossroad is the General Greene Inn, originally Bogart's Tavern. It was renamed in honor of General Nathanael Greene whose headquarters were there for a time during the Revolution. The first meeting of the Bucks County Committee for Safety was held there on July 21, 1775. The wooden sign, adorned with the General's portrait, no longer hangs in front of the inn but it may be seen inside.

From Buckingham the change in elevation is noticeable as our road descends toward Neshaminy Creek.

A few miles beyond Neshaminy Creek our road enters

Hartsville, originally known as the Cross Roads. It is a quiet hamlet extending for a mile or more along the Old York Road. On the left is the Bothwell House or "Headquarters" as it is better known. This was the headquarters of General Washington from August 10th to the 23rd, 1777, and the entire army of between twelve and thirteen thousand men camped in the nearby fields. Here also the Marquis de Lafayette was sworn in by General Washington as an officer of the Continental Army. Like so many historically important places this famous house was for many years allowed to deteriorate, but restoration during recent years has once again made it an impressive Colonial landmark.

A short distance below the "Headquarters" is a private home that was at one time a tavern known as "The Golden Glow Inn." Originally a mill, the building still retains its charm. In our research we found much conflicting information. One source, perhaps with tongue in cheek, told us that the designation "golden glow" was derived from the fact that a few glasses of the liquid cheer served at the bar gave the patrons a golden glow. We doubted the accuracy of that source and were happy to learn later that the name was in fact derived from the mass of willow trees in the yard that make a golden glow against the skies. Despite the good volume of traffic on this part of the road, the entire length of the village always seems, at least on week days, an oasis of quiet so typical of this part of Bucks County.

In the center of the village the Old York Road is crossed by the Easton-Bristol road and its original name was "the Cross Roads." John Hart, who emigrated from Whitney in Oxfordshire, England, purchased a thousand acres of land from William Penn, half of which was in Warminster, in-

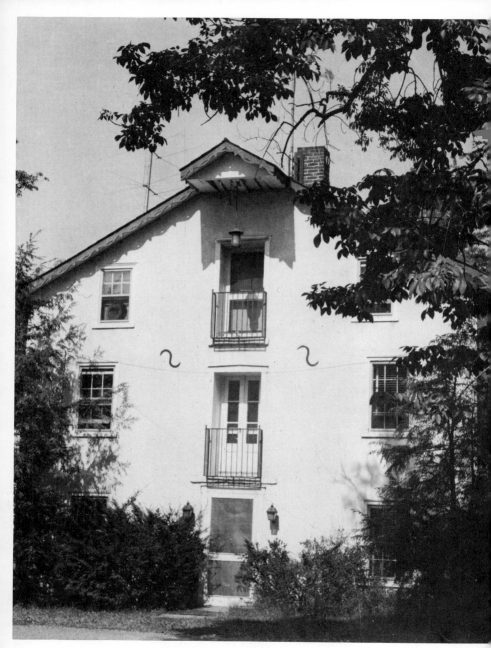

The former Golden Glow Tavern at Hartsville, now a private residence.

cluding the area that later became Cross Roads, later Hartsville. There is some confusion about when the first tavern was built. It seems, however, that the village was named for Colonel William Hart, the second son of James Hart of Plumstead Township, who moved there sometime before the middle of the eighteenth century. It is believed that the first tavern may have been the little building on the right side of the road that is now a gift shop. Other sources indicate that the north end of the present tavern, the oldest part of the building, was actually the first tavern. Whether the first tavern was built by a Hart is not clear.

Cutting through a considerable amount of conflicting information, it is believed that John Baldwin was the first owner in 1748 and probably he built the tavern. It was sold successfully to James Vansant and Colonel William Hart

The Sign of the Hart at Hartsville was built to serve travelers over both the York and Bristol Roads.

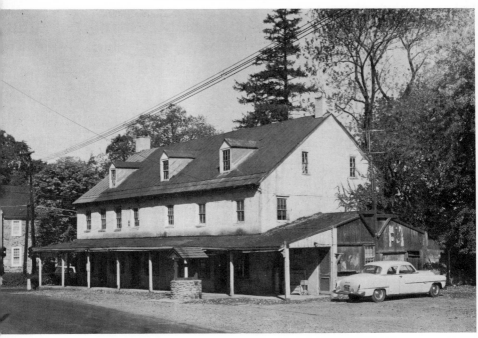

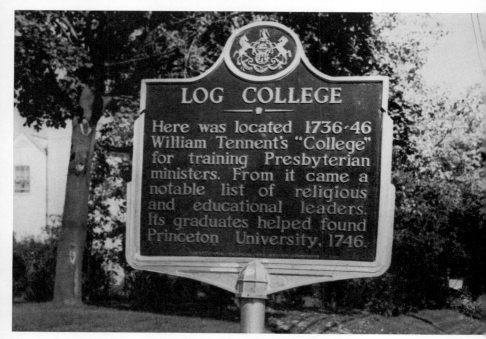

A state marker on the Old York Road commemorates one of the pioneer educational institutions of Colonial America.

who named it "The Sign of the Hart" or "The Sign of the Heart." The tavern sign had a human heart painted on it.

A state historic marker, down the road a short distance, marks the former site of the "Log College." Graduates of this humble establishment later founded many of our great American colleges. Founded in 1716 by the Reverend William Tennent, this early educational institution was housed in a log cabin. Among the great colleges that stemmed from the efforts of some of the graduates of the Log College were Princeton University, Dickenson College of Carlisle, The University of Pennsylvania, Washington University, and Hampden-Sidney College. Governor Martin of North Carolina, John Bayard, a Speaker of the House of Representatives, and many other illustrious men were among its graduates.

When the monument to the Log College was dedicated in 1889, the President of the United States, Benjamin Harrison, journeyed to Hartsville to participate in the ceremonies.

Beyond this point the former rural aspect of our road has been subjected to great changes. New shopping centers, a large parochial school and other modern buildings have been built. Warminster and Hatboro are practically one community now and both are growing rapidly as part of the Philadelphia suburban area.

In Hatboro is the old public library, believed to be the third oldest in Pennsylvania and the twelfth in the nation. It was founded in 1775 and in it today is a great repository of valuable source material for those interested in the history of Pennsylvania.

A Bucks County barn, typical of the early Pennsylvania farm buildings. The upper space was supported by stone foundations with tapered stone columns, providing implement storage at ground level.

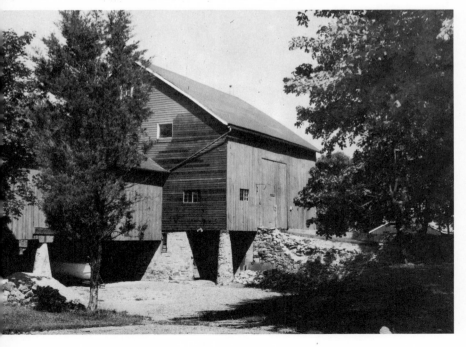

In a small plot of ground on Jacksonville Road are buried the men who died in the battle of Crooked Billet. Near the end of the village is the former grist mill, the Pennypack Mill built in 1724, and now a favored restaurant.

The town of Hatboro was originally known as Billet. This was changed to Hatboro in 1740 and was so named in honor of John Dawson who came here from England to set up a hat factory.

On a pond not far from Hatboro, below Dansville, John Fitch conducted his early experiments in the invention of a steamboat in 1785 but his inability to raise capital forced him to abandon his plans. He did, however, successfully build and run steam-propelled craft on the Delaware River before giving up his dreams. Many years later, as every school child knows, Robert Fulton carried on his experiments, copied, it is believed, from Fitch and it was he, not Fitch,

The Hatboro Library.

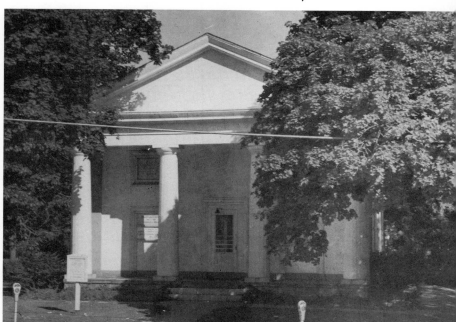

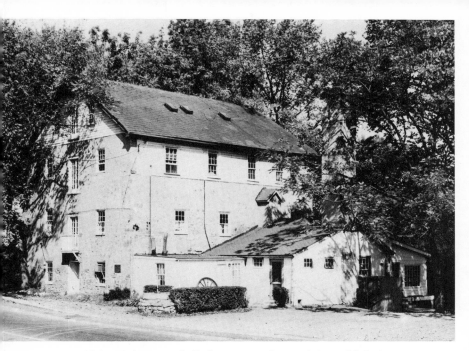

Pennypack Mill in Hatboro was built in 1724, and named for a chief of the Lenni-Lenape Indians.

who received the credit for being the inventor of the steam-boat.

It is still possible to follow the original route of the Old York Road through Willow Grove, Abington, Jenkinstown, and through Philadelphia as far as the Roosevelt Boulevard, but it is best to conclude a journey over this historic highway at Hatboro.

It is appropriate to close this narrative with a whimsical verse written at the close of the stagecoach era on our famous highway:

> And the old pike's left to die,
> The grass creeps o'er the flinty path,
> And the stealthy daisies steal,

Where once the stage horse, day by day
Lifted his iron heel.
And the old pike is left alone,
And the stages seek the plow;
We have circled the earth with an iron rail
And the steam king rules us now.

Bibliography

The works listed herein speak eloquently of the help the authors have received from writers of an earlier day. A great deal of research has been necessary to gather the material for this book. To single out and personally and properly thank all the librarians and friends who have been so generous with their time and knowledge, or to acknowledge the diaries, newspapers, and other sources would be impossible. We extend our sincere thanks to the many who have been so helpful.

Battle, J. H., *History of Bucks County, Pennsylvania.* Philadelphia, A. Warner & Co., 1887.

Cawley, James S., *Historic New Jersey in Pictures.* Princeton, Princeton University Press.

Davis, Rev. T. E., *First Houses of Bound Brook.* Bound Brook, Washington Camp Ground Association, 1893.

Davis, W. W., *History of Bucks County, Pennsylvania.* Doylestown, 1876.

Farris, John T., *Old Trails and Roads in Pennsylvania.* Philadelphia, J. B. Lippincott Co., 1927.

Harrington, M. R., *The Indians of New Jersey.* New Brunswick, Rutgers University Press, 1963.

Hart, Val, *The Story of American Roads.* New York, William Sloane Associates, 1950.

Hoff, F. Wallace, *Two Hundred Miles on the Delaware.* Trenton, The Brandt Press, 1893.

Hotchkin, Rev. S. F., *The York Road Old and New.* Philadelphia, Binder & Kelly Co., 1892.

Kalm, Peter, *The America of 1750; Travels in North America*, ed. by A. B. Benson. New York, 1937; text of English version of 1770, revised from original Swedish.

Lane, Wheaton J., *From Indian Trail to Iron Horse*. Princeton, Princeton University Press, 1939.

Larison, Cornelius, *A Country Doctor*. Trenton, New Jersey Agricultural Society, 1953.

Lathrop, Elise, *Early American Inns and Taverns*. New York, Robert M. McBride Co., Inc., 1926.

MacReynolds, George, *Place Names in Bucks County, Pennsylvania*. Doylestown, Bucks County Historical Society, 1942.

Mellick, Andrew D., Jr., *Lesser Crossroads: The Story of an Old Farm*, ed. by Hubert G. Schmidt. New Brunswick, Rutgers University Press, 1948.

Messler, Rev. A., *First Things in Old Somerset*. Somerville, Somerville Publishing Company, 1899.

Mott, George S., "First Century of Hunterdon County" (paper read before the New Jersey Historical Society, Trenton, 1878).

Quaife, Milo M.; Weig, Melvin J.; Appleman, Roy E., *The History of the United States Flag*. New York, Harper & Brothers, 1961.

Quarrie, George, *Within a Jersey Circle*. Somerville, Unionist-Gazette Association, 1910.

Perry, Charlotte Stryker, *The Bucks County Scrapbook of Old Roads and Towns*. Doylestown, privately printed, 1948.

Petrie, Alfred G., *Lambertville, New Jersey, from the Beginning as Coryell's Ferry*. Lambertville, privately printed, 1949.

Pratt, Richard A., *A Treasury of Early American Homes*. New York, Whittlesey House-McGraw Hill Book Co., 1946.

Schmidt, Hubert G., *Rural Hunterdon*. New Brunswick, Rutgers University Press, 1945.

Snell, James P., *History of Hunterdon and Somerset Counties, New Jersey*. Philadelphia, Everts & Peck, 1881.

Van Sickle, Emogene, *The Old York Road and Its Stage Coach Days*. Flemington, N.J., D. H. Moreau, 1936, 1960.

Wildes, Harry Emerson, *The Delaware*. Rivers of America Series. New York, Rinehart and Company, 1940.

146